# VETERANS

## Surviving and Thriving after Trauma

A REPRODUCIBLE WORKBOOK

CREATED FOR FACILITATORS TO USE

WITH RETURNING VETERANS

AND THEIR FAMILIES

**Ester R.A. Leutenberg & Carol Butler,** MS Ed, RN, C

Illustrations by **Amy L. Brodsky,** LISW-S
Foreword by **John Sippola,** LTC, ret., MDiv

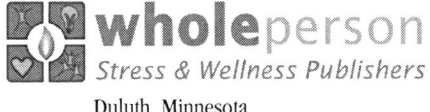

*wholeperson*
*Stress & Wellness Publishers*

Duluth, Minnesota

**Whole Person**
101 W. 2nd St., Suite 203
Duluth, MN 55802
800-247-6789

books@wholeperson.com
www.wholeperson.com

**Veterans – Surviving and Thriving After Trauma**
A reproducible workbook created for facilitators to use with returning veterans and their families

Copyright ©2013 by Ester R.A. Leutenberg and Carol Butler, MS Ed, RN, C. All rights reserved. Except for short excerpts for review purposes and materials in the assessment, journaling activities, and educational handouts sections, no part of this book may be reproduced or transmitted in any form by any means, electronic or mechanical without permission in writing from the publisher. All chapter pages with the exception of the Facilitator's Guide are meant to be photocopied.

All efforts have been made to ensure accuracy of the information contained in this book as of the date published. The author(s) and the publisher expressly disclaim responsibility for any adverse effects arising from the use or application of the information contained herein.

Printed in the United States of America

10 9 8 7 6 5 4 3 2 1

Editorial Director: Carlene Sippola
Art Director: Joy Morgan Dey

Library of Congress Control Number: 2012950509
ISBN: 978-1-57025-269-3

# *Dedication to Veterans*

Willing to
Forego familiar for foreign
Fight for freedom
Serve and save
Suffer scars
Protect us
Risk death and devastation
Return and regroup

**And to those who perished protecting their country and each other.**

**And to those whose skills sustained soldiers behind front lines.**

**And to those who help mend their wounds.**

**And to the loved ones recognized in John Milton's words:**
*They also serve who only stand and wait.*

~~~~~~~~~~~~~~~~~~~~~~~~~~~~~~~~~~~~~~~~~~~~~~~~~~~~~~~~~~

**Our gratitude to these professionals for their input ...**
Suzanne Ball, RN, BSN
Maralynn R. Bernstein
John Sippola, LTC, Ret., MDiv
Helene A. Showalter, LCSW

**And to these professionals who make us look good!**
Art Director – Joy Dey
Editor – Eileen Regen
Editorial Director – Carlene Sippola
Illustrator – Amy L. Brodsky
Proof-reader – Jay Leutenberg

~~~~~~~~~~~~~~~~~~~~~~~~~~~~~~~~~~~~~~~~~~~~~~~~~~~~~~~~~~

*Ester and Carol*

# Foreword

War casts a long shadow. For far too many service members and their families, the initial expressions of welcome, joy and relief are soon overshadowed by hidden wounds to mind, body and spirit. Too many veterans find they are engaged in yet another desperate battle. And, in this hidden war after the war they discover enemies they feel ill-equipped to fight. Aftershocks of war-related trauma and dangerous undertows of depression sabotage their mission for a more satisfying life in community. Moral injury drowns the quest for inner peace, and substance abuse undermines hard-won gains.

This workbook addresses all these challenges and more and will help you equip veterans with the skills, tools and insights they need to fight this inner war and flourish.

This book also speaks veteran vernacular, and veterans using these exercises will immediately sense fluency with military terminology that grabs their attention, inspires confidence, and puts them at ease.

Practitioners will appreciate the treasure trove of wisdom that will have them returning to this practical resource again and again.

— John Sippola, Chaplain, LTC, ret., MDiv

# Purpose of the Book

*Veterans – Surviving and Thriving after Trauma* will assist professional facilitators to help veterans adapt after serving their country. Veterans risked life, limbs, relationships and careers, some lost one or more of these basic life support systems. They freed others, but fight the aftermath of death and destruction. Many suffer emotional and physical scars, guilt, grief and loss. Some are eaten away by anger or enslaved by substances.

Initially, homecoming is happiness, applause and affection, but reintegration to daily life does not resume as they knew it. Veterans, their partners and families have changed. The labor market may not welcome their skills; their finances may plunge. Statistics show alarmingly high suicide and unemployment rates.

Help abounds via the Department of Veterans' Affairs, Department of Defense, Wounded Warrior Project and numerous governmental and private agencies. Many veterans are reluctant to seek assistance due to the perceived stigma of asking for help; others are too overwhelmed, unaware of available resources, or receive little or no help for other reasons.

As more veterans return from combat, society is increasingly aware of their needs. They will be directed toward professional and spiritual counselors. Veterans differ from other abuse survivors; they have seen atrocities and experienced horrors most civilians cannot comprehend. Their intelligence, determination and resilience that served our country are now needed to save themselves, to heal their invisible and visible wounds.

The *Veterans – Surviving and Thriving after Trauma* workbook will help facilitators working with veterans:
- Individually
- In groups
- In conjunction with their partners or families

The book's goal is for participants to ...
- realize they are not alone facing fears, feelings and challenges.
- re-integrate, as changed people, into their families and civilian life.
- deal with trauma, stress, depression, guilt and grief.
- overcome anger and resentment.
- prevent or begin recovering from substance abuse.
- handle relationship issues.
- rebound and rehabilitate emotionally, physically, vocationally, and spiritually.
- cope, using cognitive, creative, expressive, altruistic and other modes.

Veterans with or without serious emotional, physical, relationship and financial problems will benefit from the exercises which apply to the many challenges they face.

Research indicates cognitive therapy helps veterans deal with trauma and helps them improve their lives. The activities focus directly on recognizing and changing distorted ideas. Veterans see how thoughts affect feelings and actions. They are encouraged to think and act as survivors, to empower themselves to thrive despite setbacks or losses.

# For the Facilitator: Using This Book

## Format

- Description of ten topics, page vii, plus resources, pages 159–163.

- Thirty-two chapters with a Facilitator's Guide and from one to seven reproducible pages for each.

- A cover page for each topic explaining what veterans will gain from participating, a meaningful illustration, and a pertinent quotation highlighting the theme. These may be reproduced and distributed to veterans as part of an introduction to the sessions.

- Titled chapters for each topic.

- Each chapter includes the following material:
    1. **Facilitator's Guide** – the first page is for the facilitator only, to be read before the sessions. Each chapter can be divided into more than one session depending on time and participants' input.
    2. **Reproducible pages** – all of the pages with the exception of the facilitator's guide are for the participants and are reproducible. Changes can be made for a specific population by whiting out words or phrases, writing in data for the particular group and photocopying.
    3. **Education and Assessment** – activities for participants to gather personal information and to engage in self-examination.
    4. **Insight and Empowerment** – exercises to promote coping skills.

Participants are encouraged to keep the reproducible pages, their responses, art work and other exercises in three ring binders; extra notebook paper will be needed.

**The Facilitator's Guide (the first page of each chapter) has bulleted items to indicate lists of goals or interactive variation options; numbered lists are an agenda and should be followed in order.**

1. **Measurable Behavioral Objectives** show expected accomplishments.

2. **Introduction** engages interest and encourages active involvement.

3. **Activity** guides the facilitator to follow the traditional approach: reading a portion aloud, writing responses, then sharing.
    - Advise participants that where they see one line, they are to use notebook paper; they will keep the reproducible pages and their responses on lined paper in their binders.
    - Instructions direct facilitators to ask participants to share their responses.
    - Depending on the size of the group and the session's duration, there may or may not be adequate time for all participants to share all their responses.
    - If time is limited, participants may share their most important insights, or facilitators may skip to the conclusion after participants write.

4. **Conclusion** recaps and wraps up concepts discussed.

5. **Interactive Variations** provide options for talking instead of writing or working with a partner or team. Role plays and other exercises are included as appropriate.

# Topics

1. **Homecoming** – to help veterans reintegrate into families and communities and recognize that they and others have changed; to address ways to deal with partners, children and parents.

2. **Stress** – to help veterans recognize and begin to heal from emotional wounds including PTS(D), traumatic brain injury and other conditions; to emphasize cognitive changes, and mental and physical health habits.

3. **Anger** – to help veterans process issues, safely vent and express their feelings, and learn ways to de-escalate themselves and others; to highlight risks for domestic violence and safety.

4. **Depression** – to help veterans recognize signs of depression so that they can begin to heal and avoid digging deeper into despair; to incorporate hope and resilience. Sabotaging suicide is emphasized here and throughout the book.

5. **Guilt** – to help veterans decrease effects of guilt regarding death, destruction, and atrocities they were involved in or witnessed; to incorporate making amends and righting wrongs when possible.

6. **Grief** – to help veterans survive the loss of best buddies and others; to help them recognize the stages of grief and carry the torch for those they lost; to address survival guilt.

7. **Substance Abuse** – to help veterans recognize substance abuse or efforts to self-medicate with alcohol or drugs; to learn how substances intensify the spiral of ups and downs related to war's aftermath and other factors.

8. **Coping Skills** – to help veterans with cognitive, problem solving and expressive activities through art, music, writing, and other methods; to teach and emphasize relaxation techniques.

9. **Relationships** – to help veterans survive issues at home including infidelity and break-ups.

10. **Rebounding** – to help veterans deal with physical injuries and begin the process of physical healing. Options including vocational rehabilitation are included.

**Resources** – to be photocopied and distributed to all participants as one of the first introductions to this workbook. Resources refer participants to websites and agencies that help veterans and provide valuable information. On the last pages are poetry resources for facilitators who might want to suggest them to their clients. Some veterans may find these helpful; others may experience unpleasant memories. Some of the poems are graphic and facilitators might wish to read them first before recommending them to veterans.

## Safety Considerations

- Facilitators are reminded to use their experience and judgment regarding which content to present, when to present and how to present.
- Referring veterans or family members to a higher level of care is crucial if they are in danger of harming themselves or others.
- Although sessions promote coping and healing, veterans' issues may elicit explosive reactions. Facilitators should ensure that other staff members are available to work individually with participants in crisis, or to call 911 or a local Emergency Services number.

# Veterans First

Some veterans have no significant support system or do not want family involvement; therefore topics are designed for veterans. The sessions may be revised to include families, as noted below.

## Family Involvement

**Partners and family are crucial to recovery and need to be included when possible.
It is beneficial to work with veterans daily or several times a week.
It is also important to involve their partners or families in weekly multi-family sessions.**

**Confidentiality:** Veterans and partners or family members need to be aware of confidentiality; some programs ask them to sign statements regarding the rule: what happens in group stays in group.

**Room set-up:** Ideally there will be space for veterans and partners or family members to sit next to each other or in clusters, out of earshot of peers. Facilitators may need to use the hall, a patio or adjacent rooms to provide space and privacy. Facilitators can circulate among families, encouraging expression and reinforcing their efforts.

**Separate sessions first, then combine:** Some situations enable partners or families to meet first with other partners and families to share concerns, discuss the topic being addressed, and support each other; they then join their veterans for the multi-family session. Developing an educational and support group for partners and families is highly recommended.

## Ways to Involve Partners or Family

**Coaches:** The veteran's partners and/or family members read the Insight and Empowerment statements or questions to the veterans, record their responses, then share with the group if they wish. Partners may give their interpretations of the veteran's responses, validating their feelings, requesting clarification, possibly questioning perceived inaccuracies or denial.

**Helpmates:** Depending on the topic, both the veterans and family members respond to the Insight and Empowerment statements or questions in writing, then share with each other, or read them to each other and write each other's responses. They can share with the group if they wish.

**Active listening:** The veteran's partners or family members read aloud the statements or questions; the veterans respond orally; the partners reflect their feelings by paraphrasing or summarizing to show understanding. Depending on the topic, veterans may likewise read statements or questions to their partners, listen to responses, then convey comprehension.

**Practice:** Conflict resolution skills, for example, as described under the topic of 'Anger' in *De-escalation*, can be practiced by the veterans and partners, using an actual controversy they face. A third family member if present or a peer can prompt them to use the steps.

**Fishbowl:** To heighten interest and involve everyone, some veterans with their partners or families might volunteer to sit in the middle of the room, with peers in a circle around them; alternatively, they may sit in front of the room. The volunteers share written responses with each other or practice skills, (active listening, problem solving, thought changing, etc.). The onlookers, (peers), support them by giving feedback and sharing their own similar partner and family issues.

# Topics for Family Involvement

**Veterans are encouraged to share their reproducible pages and responses with their partners or family members at home.**

While any technique can include partners and families with veterans, possibilities are suggested below:

**Partners as Coaches or Active Listening:**
- Broken Bodies
- Carry the Torch
- Cognitive Counterforce Tactics
- Deception and Distortions
- Dual Battles
- Foxholes and Hope
- High Hopes for Dark Days
- Is All Fair in War?
- Nature and Nurture
- Painful or Productive Guilt?
- Post Traumatic Stress Disorder
- Reconnaissance and Resilience
- Reintegration
- Retrain Your Brain
- Romancing or Recovering?
- Sabotage Suicide
- Shock and Awe
- Shoot and Scoot
- Surviving a Breakup
- Swarming
- Vocational Rehabilitation

**Helpmates or Active Listening:**
- Anguish and Anger
- Coping and Calming A to Z
- Inducing or Reducing Anger?
- Infidelity and Introspection
- Risks for Domestic Violence
- Your Kids and Your Parents

**Practice or Fishbowl**
- De-escalation: Learn the Language
- Problems Can Be Opportunities

**Solitary activities to be shared optionally with partners and family members:**
- Art Activities
- Express Yourself
- The Mighty Pen

# Introduction for Veterans

Thank you for serving our country! You are truly welcomed home.
We are all thankful you survived.

A happy homecoming may be hampered by visible and invisible wounds. You and people close to you may have changed drastically. You may need help to heal and to re-connect.

You may be dealing with one or many of the following: reintegration, stress, anger, depression, guilt, grief, substance abuse, coping, relationships, and rebounding emotionally and physically in the aftermath of combat.

Fortunately, the bravery and resilience that sustained you during your service can help you now to survive and thrive. Fighting current battles requires a different type of combat and strategies. You have, or can develop, weapons to win the war within. You will need to tap into internal strengths and external resources.

Some veterans view seeking help as a stigma or a sign of weakness; others see it as a sign of strength. As you experience the sessions, be an active warrior. The greater your efforts, the better the pay-off. Listen with an open mind; think for yourself; feel free to respectfully disagree. Take your time; read and write thoughtfully; express your feelings.

We suggest that you keep a three ring binder for the handouts and stock plenty of notebook paper; where you see one line on your Insight and Empowerment pages, use lined paper and elaborate fully.

Remember, this is not school. When writing or drawing, don't worry about grammar, spelling or artistic talent. The work is for your eyes only unless you wish to share with peers and family. Work through the process of free expression, inspiration and recovery.

*A hero is an ordinary individual who finds the strength to persevere and endure in spite of overwhelming obstacles.*

~ Christopher Reeve

---

*Facilitators and veterans are to be applauded for working toward reintegration and recovery.*
*You are our heroes!*

Ester and Carol

# Table of Contents

1. **Homecoming**
   - Reintegration .................................................. 14–19
   - Your Kids and Your Parents ...................................... 20–24
2. **Stress**
   - PTS(D): Post Traumatic Stress (Disorder) ........................ 26–29
   - Coping and Calming A to Z ....................................... 30–33
   - Deception and Distortions ....................................... 34–38
   - Shoot and Scoot ................................................. 39–43
   - Swarming ........................................................ 44–45
   - Re-Train Your Brain ............................................. 46–49
3. **Anger**
   - Anguish and Anger ............................................... 52–57
   - De-escalation: Learn the Language ............................... 58–61
   - Inducing or Reducing Anger? ..................................... 62–64
   - Risks for Domestic Violence ..................................... 65–68
4. **Depression**
   - High Hopes and Dark Days ........................................ 70–73
   - Foxholes and Hope ............................................... 74–77
   - Reconnaissance and Resilience ................................... 78–81
   - Sabotage Suicide ................................................ 82–87
5. **Guilt**
   - Is All Fair in War? ............................................. 90–92
   - Painful or Productive Guilt? .................................... 93–95
6. **Grief**
   - Shock and Awe ................................................... 98–101
   - Carry the Torch ................................................. 102–103
7. **Substance Abuse**
   - Nature and Nurture .............................................. 106–109
   - Romancing or Recovering? ........................................ 110–112
   - Dual Battles .................................................... 113–116
8. **Coping Skills**
   - Cognitive Counterforce Tactics .................................. 118–124
   - Problems Can Be Opportunities ................................... 125–129
   - Art Activities .................................................. 130–133
   - The Mighty Pen (Journaling) ..................................... 134–136
   - Express Yourself ................................................ 137–139
9. **Relationships**
   - Infidelity and Introspection .................................... 142–143
   - Surviving a Breakup ............................................. 144–147
10. **Rebounding**
    - Broken Bodies .................................................. 150–155
    - Vocational Rehabilitation ...................................... 156–158

**Resources**
   - Web-Site Resources for Veterans ................................. 160
   - Books for Veterans and Families ................................. 161
   - Additional Internet Search Topics ............................... 162
   - Suggestions for Veterans and/or Veterans' Families at the Facilitator's Discretion .. 163

# Homecoming

*Returning home is the most difficult part of long-distance hiking;*
*You have grown outside the puzzle and your piece no longer fits.*

~ Cindy Ross

Re-entering civilian life and re-connecting with family and friends can be both a negative and positive experience for veterans coming home. Homecoming will help veterans identify relationship changes, invisible wounds, needs, challenges, a rationale for hope, and new ways to think. They will focus on improving communication and reestablishing their relationship with their children, partners, parents, family and friends.

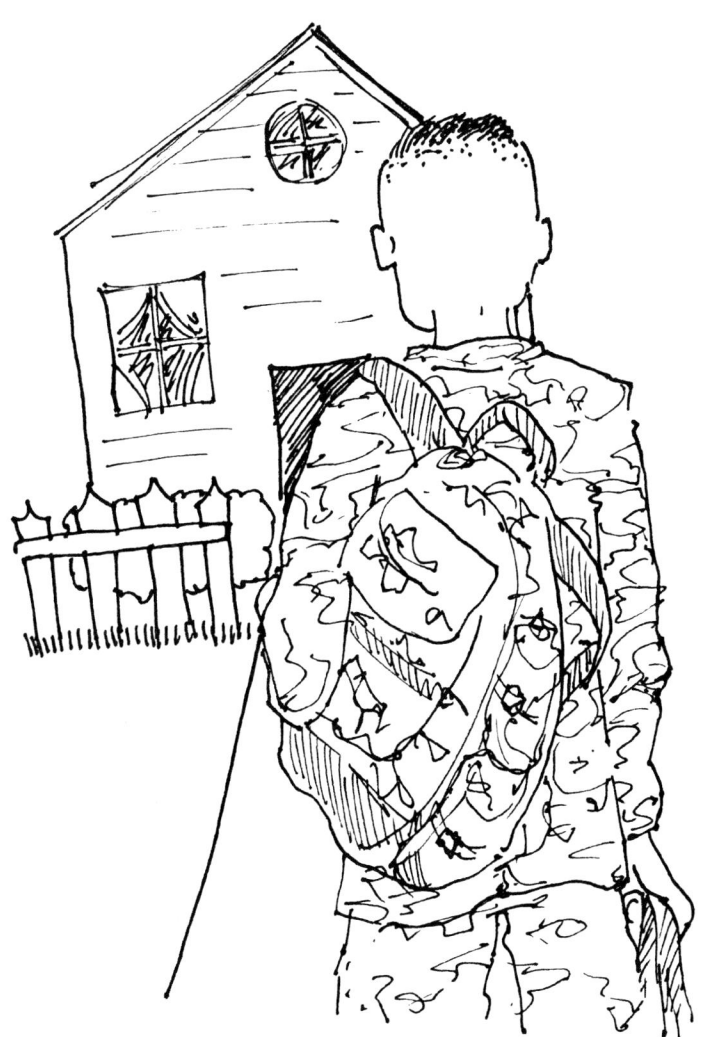

VETERANS: SURVIVING AND THRIVING AFTER TRAUMA

# Reintegration Facilitator's Guide

## Measurable Behavioral Objectives
**Veterans will …**
- Rate themselves regarding responses to post-deployment and re-entry issues.
- Recognize reasons to seek help and resources for professional treatment.
- State their top immediate needs, emotions and challenges.
- Answer questions to elicit cognitive and behavioral changes and instill hope.
- Discuss invisible wounds and what they are doing or will do to help them heal.
- Describe the top qualities of winners, in war and civilian life.

## Introduction
1. Before the session begins, read this guide and the reproducible pages.
2. Decide on one of the interactive variations or the traditional approach (below).
3. Photocopy the reproducible pages but retain them until after the introduction.
4. Put the word *Homecoming* on the board and ask participants to compare how they thought homecoming would be compared to the reality of their homecoming experiences.
5. Put the word *Reintegration* on the board and ask participants to brainstorm aspects of resuming daily life.
6. Ask for a volunteer to list the ideas on the board.
7. Explain that this exercise will help everyone to consider ways to cope with the radical changes from military service life to civilian life.

## Activity
1. Distribute the reproducible pages.
2. Take turns reading the Education and Assessment portion aloud.
3. Encourage participants to check the applicable items as they are read.
4. Allow time to complete the written Insight and Empowerment questions.
5. Encourage group members to share their answers through number 20.

## Conclusion
- Encourage participants to share at least one of their responses to the quotations (numbers 21 and 22).
- Ask group members to share other military quotes they have heard, or to make up their own words of wisdom regarding reintegration.

## Interactive Variations
- Ask participants to take turns reading aloud the Insight and Empowerment questions and answering orally.
- Ask them to pair up with peers, read the questions to each other, record their partner's responses, then share with the group if they wish.

EDUCATION AND ASSESSMENT

# Reintegration

**Although you left combat, the war is probably still with you.**
**Reintegration, being a civilian again, means a new normal; life may never be the same as you once knew it.**

**Check the items that you are experiencing. Add your unique responses on the blank lines:**
- ❑ I had or am having a wonderful honeymoon phase.
- ❑ I am appreciated for my patriotism.
- ❑ People recognize my new skills, maturity, and other attributes.
- ❑ I am a positive role model for my children.
- ❑ My family bonds are strengthened.
- ❑ My flexibility and adaptation to change benefit myself and others.
- ❑ I am able to re-negotiate rules and roles better after I have been home a while.
- ❑ I re-evaluate my relationship, and its goals, and the direction it will take.
- ❑ I am grateful I am a survivor.
- ❑ I feel a roller-coaster of emotions.
- ❑ I will never be the same.
- ❑ People do not understand what I have been through and how I have changed.
- ❑ I question whether people will accept the new me.
- ❑ I need time and space and resent probing questions by well-meaning people.
- ❑ My homecoming is not what I expected.
- ❑ My reception seemed lukewarm.
- ❑ It is difficult to re-connect with my partner emotionally or physically.
- ❑ My transition from being single to a couple is difficult.
- ❑ My relationship and roles are changing because my partner and I have changed.
- ❑ I am engaged in power struggles.
- ❑ I encounter resistance as I try to resume my prior authority or role.
- ❑ My parents still treat me like a child.
- ❑ My children may remain detached because they fear another separation.
- ❑ The kids fear my discipline; my partner warned, "Just wait until daddy or mommy gets home!"
- ❑ Teens rebel against my rules and expectations.
- ❑ I expect schedules and regimentation; my family is undisciplined; my home disorganized.
- ❑ I miss contact with veterans who have *been there and done that*.
- ❑ My partner does not understand my need to stay connected with buddies.
- ❑ I feel survivor's guilt because I lived and some of my buddies died.
- ❑ I dislike the whirlwind of welcoming activities.
- ❑ I think it is too soon for household chores, school, or work; but feel the pressure.
- ❑ I find it hard to do my old job.
- ❑ I cannot get work; employers do not value my skills.
- ❑ I am the supposed to be hero, but others want credit for responsibilities handled at home or work.
- ❑ I am concerned about future or multiple deployments.
- ❑ _____
- ❑ _____
- ❑ _____
- ❑ _____

EDUCATION AND ASSESSMENT

# Give Yourself Hope

**Check the items you agree with or hope to eventually believe:**

- ❑ Many experiences do evoke sorrow, regret, anger, rebellion and determination to change conditions.
- ❑ These feelings and thoughts need not evolve into depression, worthlessness, rage and panic.
- ❑ Something that once strongly affected my life need not indefinitely or forever ruin it.
- ❑ I do have control over my reactions now, despite my initial response to terror.
- ❑ There is not a magic cure for problems; I can seek solutions, and experiment with trial and error.
- ❑ I know people behave unjustly in war, but I can accept this without agreeing, and work to better the world.
- ❑ Conditions seem unfavorable, but I can accept what cannot be changed and change what I can change.
- ❑ I can face fearsome facts rather than avoiding or obsessing about them.
- ❑ Progress versus perfection can be achieved.
- ❑ Probability and chance exist; I can't control outcomes; I can control my thoughts, feelings and actions.
- ❑ Inertia, inaction, hopelessness and helplessness can be replaced with pursuits outside myself.
- ❑ While love and acceptance feel great, I need not seek absolute approval from everyone.
- ❑ I can act in ways that foster self-respect and are congruent with my values.
- ❑ My depression or happiness are not dependent on people or circumstances but on my thoughts.
- ❑ I can choose reliable, supportive people versus folks known to be fickle or reckless.
- ❑ I can tolerate discomfort and pain, and may be strengthened as a result.
- ❑ Mistakes are learning experiences.

Compounding routine reintegration, (usually three to seven months), you may have PTS(D), post traumatic stress disorder, TBI, traumatic brain injury, or other physical or emotional problems. Medical and psychological evaluations are required for overwhelming sadness, anger, inability to eat or sleep, severe pain, and other symptoms.

**If you are thinking about suicide, with a plan and a means to carry it out, call 911 or your local Emergency Services number, the National Suicide Prevention Lifeline/Veteran's Crisis Line, 1-800-273-8255 (TALK), or go to your nearest hospital Emergency Room.**

INSIGHT AND EMPOWERMENT

# Combat to Civilian: From Foreign War Zone to Homefront Battles

Place a check by the statement that best describes your re-entry. Then elaborate in the fourth column.

| Reality of Service | Re-entry Goals | Re-entry Battles | Elaborate: Which are you right now? |
|---|---|---|---|
| *Ex: From a military might* | *to a civilian identity* | *to not fitting in* ✔ | *I don't feel as if I fit in anywhere.* |
| Reality of danger | to safety | to new fears | |
| Uncomfortable conditions | to comfort | to different discomforts | |
| Camaraderie | to other types of companionship | to loneliness | |
| Mistrust | to trust | to new suspicions | |
| Chaos | to order | to confusion | |
| Following orders | to making my own decisions | to indecisiveness | |
| Acting first and thinking later | to contemplation and planning | to impulsivity | |
| Numbing emotions | to express emotions | to hide or displace emotions | |
| Adrenaline rushes | to peace | to boredom or heightened anxiety | |
| A life or death job | to a satisfying role | to meaninglessness | |
| Regimentation | to flexibility and choice | to aimlessness | |

## INSIGHT AND EMPOWERMENT
# What You Can Do Now

1. List your top five immediate needs and your plan to share them with your partner or family.

   _____
   _____
   _____
   _____
   _____
   _____

2. Describe a situation that elicits emotions within you.

   _____

3. What can you tell yourself to prevent the situation and feelings from severely depressing you?

   _____

4. What will you say to yourself to prevent the past from ruining your present and future?

   _____

5. Think about a situation that led to sadness. What do you now know that can prevent continued despair?

   _____

6. Describe a valuable lesson you learned from a mistake:

   _____

7. Regarding other people's destructive or ignorant behavior: What can you tell yourself to prevent rage?

   _____

8. What potentially unpleasant facts must you currently accept?

   _____

9. What potentially unpleasant circumstances can you change?

   _____

10. What scary situations would be helpful to face rather than avoid or obsess about?

    _____

11. Regardless of the outcome, what will you tell yourself after you face your fears?

    _____

12. Praise yourself for progress concerning a current problem, versus condemning yourself for imperfection.

    _____

*(Continued on the next page)*

## INSIGHT AND EMPOWERMENT

# What You Can Do Now *(Continued)*

13. Describe your experience with bad luck. What will you tell yourself about your ability to control events?

14. What can you do to right a wrong regarding social injustice, a mistake, or conditions you dislike?

15. If you feel sad or unloved, how can you make someone happy or show your concern or affection?

16. Why can you not expect everyone, or your loved ones, to approve of everything you say or do?

17. Share a current conflict where you are acting on your belief system despite disapproval from others:

18. How can you keep yourself upbeat in a current situation where people or circumstances let you down?

19. Share a thought that has made your military experience seem worse:

20. Change the thought to a positive but realistic alternative:

21. ***In war there are no unwounded soldiers.*** ~ Jose Narosky.

    This refers to invisible wounds. Share thoughts about your wounds and what you are doing, or will do, to help heal them.

22. ***Wars may be fought with weapons, but they are won by men.*** ~ General George Patton Jr.

    Describe the top five qualities that make men and women, including you, winners in war and life:

# Your Kids and Your Parents Facilitator's Guide

## Measurable Behavioral Objectives
**Veterans will …**
- Identify risk factors regarding their children's adjustment.
- Recognize problems and when to seek professional help.
- Read considerations and tips to help kids during post-deployment.
- Identify sources of friendship and support for their children.
- Consider new family traditions to incorporate.
- Encourage children's self-expression using art, journaling, or two other methods.
- Elicit from their children answers about the advantages of military life.
- Apply insightful quotations to themselves and their children.
- Answer questions to help handle their parents' expectations and concerns.

## Introduction
1. Before the session read this guide and the reproducible pages.
2. Decide on one of the interactive activities or the traditional approach (below).
3. Photocopy the reproducible pages but retain them until after the introduction.
4. Ask group members to brainstorm how youngsters are affected by their parent's homecoming.
5. You or a volunteer participant will list ideas on the board.
6. Ask participants to brainstorm the positive qualities kids from military families develop.
7. A volunteer lists them on the board.
8. Explain that they will address handling homecoming with kids and issues regarding their parents.

## Activity
1. Distribute the reproducible pages.
2. Take turns reading the Education and Assessment portion aloud.
3. Encourage participants to check the applicable boxes as they read.
4. Allow time to complete the written Insight and Empowerment questions.
5. Encourage them to share their answers through number 6.

## Conclusion
- Encourage participants to share their responses to the quotations (numbers 7-10).
- Encourage participants to share answers to the Relationship with Your Parents questions.

## Interactive Variations
- Ask participants to take turns reading the Insight and Empowerment questions aloud and answering orally.
- Ask participants to pair up with peers, read the questions to each other, record their partner's responses, then share with the group if they wish.

EDUCATION AND ASSESSMENT

# Your Kids and Your Parents

## About Children . . .

- Children whose parents suffer after combat are at risk for emotional problems.
- Reassuring youngsters they are loved and will be cared for helps them adjust.
- Kids often mimic parental moods and behavior.
- Parenting classes on bases and in communities provide helpful tips and support.
- Children and the family need professional help if a parent has physical, emotional or addiction problems, or if domestic violence or child abuse is imminent.
- If your child wants to harm him/herself or others, call 911 or your local Emergency Services number or go to the nearest hospital's Emergency Room.

## Your child loves you but homecoming brings changes:

- Respect your children's maturation and growth that occurred in your absence.
- Avoid suddenly taking an overly authoritarian role.
- Plan discipline, rules and responsibilities that both parents agree upon.
- You can set up calendars, charts, checklists, sticker systems for young children, and other rewards for teens.
- Keep up with schoolwork; inform teachers and counselors you have returned.
- Seek activities, clubs, sports, house of worship youth groups, camps, for the kids.
- Find enjoyable things to do as a family.
- Expect reunification to take time, versus instant warm-fuzzy feelings.

INSIGHT AND EMPOWERMENT

# Warning signs indicating that children may need professional help

Check the boxes that apply to your **toddler(s)**:
- ❑ Clingy, tearful, more temper tantrums
- ❑ Regression such as wanting a bottle after weaning; more toileting accidents
- ❑ Changes in sleep, wakefulness, nightmares; considerable change in food intake
- ❑ Keeping parent always in sight; more fearful of new people or situations

Check the boxes that apply to your **school age child(ren)**:
- ❑ Regression, any of the above behaviors
- ❑ Unsubstantiated physical complaints, headaches, stomach problems
- ❑ Irritability, anger at little things, fighting at school, grumpy at home
- ❑ Decline in grades
- ❑ Loss of interest in previously enjoyed activities

Check the boxes that apply to your **teen(s)**:
- ❑ Regression, any of the above behaviors
- ❑ Decreased self-esteem
- ❑ Isolation, withdrawal
- ❑ Signs or symptoms of anxiety, depression, adjustment problems
- ❑ Substance abuse

1. Your own mental health is most crucial to your children's well-being. State at least three things you are doing to help yourself cope such as professional help if needed, having a support system, keeping yourself physically and mentally healthy, using positive thinking:
   _____
   _____

2. State at least three things you are doing to help your kids find friendship and support:
   _____
   _____

3. Identify current rituals and family traditions; state at least two new ones to add:
   _____
   _____

4. Encourage self-expression through young children's play: get down on the floor, use dolls, stuffed animals, toy vehicles; go with the flow of the youngsters' fantasies; make available music and art for all ages, and journaling for older kids. What opportunities have you provided and how can you add at least two more avenues for sharing feelings?
   _____
   _____

5. *A picture is worth a thousand words*, especially to young children or withdrawn teens. Encourage drawing, then let them talk about the picture; fears and anger may emerge. Ask them to depict their family. Notice who is big, small, who is near whom, facial expressions, and other clues. What have your children revealed through their explanations of their art?
   _____
   _____

INSIGHT AND EMPOWERMENT

# Accentuate the Positives

**Military children benefit. Help them identify their blessings.**

1. They have broader experiences. Ask them to share things they have done and places they have been that others their age rarely encounter. What answers do you expect or will you elicit?
   _____
   _____

2. Military youngsters develop social skills, must frequently make new friends, and face goodbyes. Ask them what people skills they have developed from frequent relocations. What answers do you expect or will you elicit?
   _____
   _____

3. Ask them how they have changed due to more responsibilities. What answers do you expect or will you elicit?
   _____
   _____

4. Ask them about the interests and abilities they developed due to their military involvement. What answers do you expect or will you elicit?
   _____
   _____

5. Your children are likely to be independent self-starters. Ask them for examples they see in themselves or how they plan to practice this skill. What answers do you expect or will you elicit?
   _____
   _____

6. Family bonds may strengthen due to military experience. Ask them how your family is closer. What answers do you expect or will you elicit?
   _____
   _____

7. ***Don't worry that your children never listen to you; worry that they are always watching you.*** ~ Robert Fulghum. What do you want your children to see in you?
   _____
   _____

8. ***Your children need your presence more than your presents.*** ~ Jesse Jackson.
   How are you going to be available mentally and provide quality time?
   _____
   _____

9. ***Don't handicap your children by making their lives easy.*** ~ Robert A. Heinlein
   What challenges are you providing to strengthen your children?
   _____
   _____

10. ***If there is anything we wish to change in the child, we should first examine it and see whether it is not something that could better be changed in ourselves.*** ~ Carl Gustav Jung.
    About which trait(s) does this apply to your child(ren) and you?
    _____
    _____

## INSIGHT AND EMPOWERMENT
# Your Relationship with Your Parents

Ways you've changed impact your relationship, especially if you are single and living with your parents. You will always be their child, yet you are more adult than ever. You risked your life for them, saw and did things they know nothing about, and matured faster than they realize. You are older than your years. Practice below by writing what you need to say to them.

1. Tell them what you need, especially about time, space, privacy or preferred frequency of family activities:

2. How will you politely refrain from answering questions? (Example: *Thanks for caring but I prefer not to talk about it now.*)

3. Be proactive; they may be concerned if you show signs of emotional, physical or substance abuse problems. What will you tell them you are doing about any of these that apply?

4. What are you doing about any other valid concerns?

5. If they were primary caregivers for your children, expect them to have mixed feelings about relinquishing their role. How will you handle resuming your parental role without breaking the strong bonds they developed during your deployment?

# Stress

*"The greatest weapon against stress is our ability to choose one thought over another."*

~ William James

**V**ETERANS WILL RATE THEMSELVES regarding post traumatic stress (disorder), traumatic brain injury, and other stress responses; they will learn and practice coping and calming skills, talk about differences between rational and irrational fears, and use cognitive therapy techniques to improve thoughts, feelings and actions. Veterans will help each other and work together to identify ways to de-stress via thought replacements and learning to re-train their brains through physical and mental health interventions.

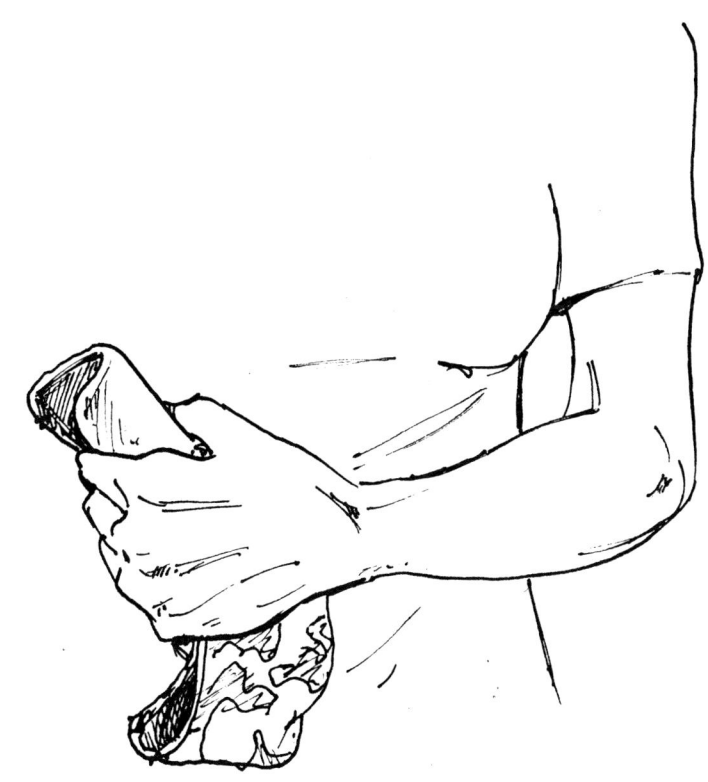

# PTS(D): Post Traumatic Stress (Disorder) Facilitator's Guide

## Measurable Behavioral Objectives
**Veterans will ...**
- Identify common responses to trauma they may have experienced.
- Rate themselves regarding PTS(D) symptoms.
- Describe their risk factors for PTS(D).
- Describe their triggers leading to extreme reactions or flashbacks.
- Share ways their PTS(D) impacts areas of their lives such as substance abuse, relationships, employment, aggression, suicidal ideation or other repercussions.
- Describe how veterans and family members can better understand and help each other heal.
- Define ways they can strengthen their spirituality to facilitate more faith, hope, joy and love.
- Analyze a thought-provoking quotation about adversity and apply it to their lives.

## Introduction
1. Before the session begins, read this guide and the reproducible pages.
2. Decide on one of the interactive variations or the traditional approach (below).
3. Photocopy the reproducible pages but retain them until after the introduction.
4. Secretly enlist a volunteer to startle peers, (drop a book or other object or to make a loud noise), as you start group.
5. Ask those who jumped or reacted to raise their hands; explain that being startled by loud noises is natural, but some people react in exaggerated ways, depending on exposure to trauma.
6. Write on the board *Responses to Trauma* and *Signs of PTS(D)*.
7. Ask participants to brainstorm while a volunteer lists their ideas on the board.
8. Explain that trauma can be from combat exposure or other horrific situations.

## Activity
1. Distribute the reproducible pages.
2. Take turns reading the Education and Assessment portion aloud.
3. Encourage participants to check the applicable boxes as they are read.
4. Allow time to complete the written Insight and Empowerment questions.
5. Encourage participants to share their answers through number 9.

## Conclusion
Encourage participants to share responses to the quotation (number 10).

## Interactive Variations
- Ask participants to take turns reading Insight and Empowerment questions aloud and answering orally.
- Ask them to pair up with peers, read the questions to each other, record their partner's responses, then share with the group if they wish.

EDUCATION AND ASSESSMENT

# PTS(D): Post Traumatic Stress (Disorder)

Exposure to combat, witnessing death and destruction and other trauma can lead to common reactions that resolve soon. When reactions persist over time they become post-trauma symptoms. Many veterans have an array of post-traumatic stress symptoms. These symptoms may not rise to the level of a formal diagnosis. Nevertheless, they may significantly hinder the joy and quality of daily living and need to be addressed.

**Check the following common responses to trauma that apply to you:**

- ❑ Anxiety, the fight or flight reaction, freezing with fear, being jumpy and watchful.
- ❑ Sadness or depression, crying, lack of interest or enjoyment, self-isolation, fatigue.
- ❑ Guilt and shame: feeling you could have done more, surviving when others did not.
- ❑ Irritable and angry about unfair treatment, low levels of patience, overreacting.
- ❑ Behavior changes, increased substance use, reckless driving, self-neglect.

**Symptoms of PTS(D)** for the person who experienced or witnessed an event involving actual or threatened death or serious injury and responded with intense fear, helplessness or horror, include the following:

**Check those that apply to you.**

- ❑ Re-experiencing or reliving the event with the same terror, images, thoughts, perceptions; dissociative flashbacks, nightmares, illusions, hallucinations.
- ❑ Intense psychological distress reaction to triggers which are internal or external cues that resemble an aspect of the trauma.
- ❑ Avoiding reminders - people, places, things such as crowds, cars if your convoy was attacked, fireworks; keeping too busy and not addressing related thoughts and feelings; and not talking about traumatic experiences.
- ❑ Numbness, feeling shut-down, detached or estranged from others; not feeling affection or joy; inability to recall aspects of the trauma; diminished interest in formerly significant activities; harboring a sense of foreshortened future, not expecting a normal life-span.
- ❑ Hyper-arousal, easily startled, poor sleep patterns; irritability or anger outbursts; hyper-vigilance, (on guard).
- ❑ Feeling lost, alone, distrustful, awkward, and afraid most of the time.
- ❑ PTS(D) disturbance causes significant distress in social, occupational or other important areas of daily functioning.

*(Continued on the next page)*

EDUCATION AND ASSESSMENT

# PTS(D): Post Traumatic Stress (Disorder)

**Factors contributing to combat-related PTS(D) include:**

- trauma's severity and duration
- relationship with the persons hurt or killed
- injury
- intensity of response
- degree of powerlessness or control
- quality and amount of help received after the event
- being shot at or physically harmed
- being sexually assaulted
- killing or injuring a fellow military person, woman, child, fellow country-person, civilian
- physically or sexually assaulting or torturing others
- harming animals
- witnessing injury or death among buddies
- seeing, smelling and handling dead bodies
- an unsuccessful rescue
- mercy killing
- involvement in property destruction and atrocities
- exposure to toxins

**Other impetuses for severe stress reaction include:**

- constant fear of injury or death
- worrying about nuclear, chemical or biological attack
- experiencing bad accidents, heat stroke, dehydration and sleep deprivation

**Veterans are at greater risk if** they had earlier trauma such as child abuse, mental illness, a family history of emotional problems, poor support system, limited education, or other recent life changes.

**PTS(D) often leads to** self-medicating through substance abuse, employment and relationship problems, hopelessness, depression, despair, shame, aggression and suicidal ideation.

**People may not seek help** due to the perceived stigma of mental illness, long waits for treatment, denial, or cultural factors such as being stoic versus false perception of weakness if asking for help.

**When family members suggest getting help** veterans are urged to follow through to respect their loved one's concerns.

**Denial is a common response** yet tough people suffer symptoms, not always combat-related. Victims of abuse, accidents and natural disasters are at also at risk.

**Physical reactions** may involve chronic pain, heart palpitations, trouble breathing, profuse perspiring, stomach upsets and other bodily reactions to anything that reminds the person of the stressful military experience.

INSIGHT AND EMPOWEREMENT)

# PTS(D): Post Traumatic Stress (Disorder)

1. What traumatic events and factors have contributed to your stress response?

2. List your most troublesome PTS(D) symptoms, if applicable:

3. What are your personal risk factors?

4. What are your triggers – sights, sounds, smells, tastes, sensations, situations and other events that cause flashbacks or extreme emotional and or physical reactions?

5. How has your life been affected by your PTS(D)? Share thoughts about substance abuse, employment, relationships, anger, aggression, suicidal ideation and/or other repercussions:

6. What treatment(s) do you think might help you? How will you access mental health care?

7. How have your loved ones/family been affected by your symptoms?

8. How can veterans and families better understand and help each other through the healing process?

9. How can you strengthen your spirituality to facilitate more faith, hope, joy and love?

10. Relate the following quote to your experience with war and trauma. Explain whether and why or how you agree or disagree:

    ***Every adversity, every failure, every heartache carries with it the seed of an equal or greater benefit.*** ~ Napoleon Hill

# Coping and Calming: A to Z Facilitator's Guide

## Measurable Behavioral Objectives

**Veterans will ...**
- Read and brainstorm ways to cope and reduce stress.
- Identify skills that best suit them and state how they will use them.
- Identify unfamiliar methods. Research and report a fact for each.
- Describe thoughts or plans regarding pets, service or therapy dogs.
- Describe how they would benefit from volunteering to help veterans or others.
- Develop A to Z list of skills.
- Apply quotations to personal experiences and thoughts related to visualization, adversity, warriors and challenges.
- Describe actions to develop their faculties, increase energy and fulfill their destiny based on a Colin Powell quotation.

## Introduction

1. Before the session begins, read this guide and the reproducible pages and decide on one of the interactive variations or the traditional approach below.
2. Photocopy the reproducible pages but retain them until after the introduction.
3. Put on the board *Coping and Calming Skills* and ask group members to brainstorm techniques.
4. You or a volunteer participant lists them on the board.

## Activity

1. Distribute the reproducible pages.
2. Take turns reading aloud the Education portion.
3. Allow time to complete the written Insight and Empowerment questions.
4. Encourage everyone to share their responses through number 5.

## Conclusion

- Encourage them to share all or their most meaningful responses to the quotations numbers 6-10.

## Interactive Variations

- Ask them to take turns reading aloud the Insight and Empowerment questions and answering them orally.
- Ask them to pair up with peers, read the questions to each other, record their partner's responses, then share with the group if they wish.

## Teams

1. Split the group into two teams; one takes letters A-L; the other takes M-Z.
2. Teams brainstorm coping and calming skills and elect a person to record them.
3. Teams reunite and share ideas.
4. Then proceed to read the reproducible pages aloud, write answers, (except for number 5), and share responses.

EDUCATION

# Coping and Calming: A to Z

**Coping with trauma or emotions such as anger, and calming yourself down when anxious or afraid requires skills. Below are some ideas for further exploration:**

Act as if you are brave when fearful.

Be aware you are now in safe surroundings.

Create calm and confident thoughts to affect feelings and actions.

Dogs help as service and therapy pets for vets.

Express personal feelings; exercise to boost endorphins, the feel-good brain chemicals.

Feed your mind with faith and forgiveness.

Go with gratitude for your survival.

Have hope for healing.

Internal focus means you control your own thoughts, actions, and destiny.

Just do the things you fear, love and can do.

Keep away the clutter in your mind and life.

Lose yourself in loved activities.

Move out of your comfort zone.

Never give up.

Open up to trusted people.

Pursue your passion and purpose.

Question your qualms.

Re-create you.

Success-oriented self-talk promotes confidence.

Take time-out if angry.

Uplift your mood with humor, fun and spirituality.

Volunteer to help others.

Walk and work-out.

X-ray vision helps you see your invisible wounds.

You control your thoughts, feelings, actions and recovery.

Zap helpless thinking.

*(Continued on the next page)*

INSIGHT AND EMPOWERMENT

# Coping and Calming: A to Z

1. Select at least five coping skills from page 31 and state how they will help, and how you will use them.
2. Select at least five concepts from the A to Z list on page 31 you would like to know more about. Ask people, or do an online search, and share at least one new fact about each.
3. Describe your thoughts or plans about getting a dog or pet for companionship and unconditional love, or for exploring service or therapy dog opportunities.
4. Describe how you can be of service by volunteering to help other veterans, or by volunteering in your community.
5. Make your own coping and calming skills list:

A - 
B - 
C - 
D - 
E - 
F - 
G - 
H - 
I - 
J - 
K - 
L - 
M - 
N - 
O - 
P - 
Q - 
R - 
S - 
T - 
U - 
V - 
W - 
X - 
Y - 
Z - 

*(Continued on the next page)*

INSIGHT AND EMPOWERMENT

# Coping and Calming: A to Z *(Continued)*

6. ***You won't see how to do it until you see yourself doing it.*** ~ David Allen
   Share your vision of you doing something you need to do for your healing so that you are better able to live life to the fullest:
   _____
   _____
   _____

7. ***Adversity has the effect of eliciting talents which, in prosperous circumstances, would have lain dormant.*** ~ Horace
   What talents are emerging or do you hope to discover from your difficulties?
   _____
   _____
   _____

8. ***The basic difference between an ordinary man and a warrior is that a warrior takes everything as a challenge while an ordinary man takes everything as a blessing or a curse.*** ~ Carlos Castaneda
   What possible curse is a challenge and in what three ways are you facing it as a warrior?
   _____
   _____
   _____

9. ***The best place to succeed is where you are with what you have.*** ~ Charles Schwab
   Describe where you are, what you have, how you will succeed, and in which endeavors:
   _____
   _____
   _____

10. ***The chief condition, on which life, health and vigor depend is action. It is by action that an organism develops its faculties, increases its energy and obtains fulfillment of its destiny.***
    ~ Colin Powell
    _____
    _____
    _____

Describe at least two specific actions for each step forward:

   a. To develop my faculties:
   _____
   _____

   b. To increase my energy:
   _____
   _____

   c. To fulfill my destiny:
   _____
   _____

VETERANS: SURVIVING AND THRIVING AFTER TRAUMA

# Deception and Distortions Facilitator's Guide

## Measureable Behavioral Goals
**Veterans will ...**
- Identify negative thoughts they often experience.
- Identify distortions, detrimental feelings and actions.
- Practice replacing distortions with positive and realistic thoughts.
- Identify the resultant more favorable feelings and actions.
- Discuss quotes about cognitive changes and apply these ideas to their own lives.

## Introduction
1. Before the session begins, read this guide and the reproducible pages.
2. Decide on one of the interactive variations or the traditional approach (below).
3. Photocopy the reproducible pages but retain them until after the introduction.
4. If available, show a label, coffee filter, magnifying glass, or a half full glass of water.
5. Ask, *"What do these items have to do with our thinking?"* Elicit responses recognizing that we label ourselves and others; look at the negatives such as used coffee grounds, filter out, ignore positive aspects; magnify problems or imperfections in ourselves; and see the glass as half-empty or deficient versus half-full with possibilities.

## Activity
1. Distribute the reproducible pages.
2. Take turns reading aloud the Education and Assessment portion.
3. Encourage participants to check applicable the boxes as they are read.
4. Take turns reading aloud the Insight and Empowerment directions and examples.
5. Allow time to complete the written questions 1-5.
6. Encourage participants to share their answers through number 5.

## Conclusion
- Write the quotations (number 6) on the board and encourage the participants to debate and discuss them.

## Interactive Variations
- Ask participants to answer all Insight and Empowerment questions orally and receive feedback. It is helpful for the facilitator to make a chart on the board for thoughts, distortions, feelings, actions and replacement thoughts, feelings and actions as participants share.
- Ask participants to pair up with peers, read the questions to each other, record their partner's responses, then share with the group if they wish.

EDUCATION AND ASSESSMENT

# Deception and Distortions

**DECEPTION** in military terms means a strategy that seeks to deceive, trick or fool the enemy and create a false perception in a way that can be leveraged for a military advantage.

**DISTORTED THOUGHTS** deceive us and make us miserable. Cognitive therapy asserts that thoughts affect feelings which affect actions.

**Example:** A service person **thinks** *I should have died when my buddy died; I'll never enjoy life again.*
> The service person **feels** depressed, guilty, hopeless and worthless.
> The service person **acts** in detrimental ways such as drinking or drugging to escape, driving recklessly, possibly attempting suicide, all because of thinking I don't deserve to live.

**Example:** A partner **thinks** the changes are very drastic: *I don't even know the person I married.*
> The partner **feels** overwhelmed, unable to understand, scared.
> The partner **acts** standoffish, fearful, irritated.

Distorted thoughts are your current enemy. They have been camouflaged but now you will recognize them.

Place a check or highlight the distortions that describe ways you usually think.

| DISTORTION | EXAMPLE |
|---|---|
| **All or Nothing or Black or White** | You see absolutes: right or wrong, good or bad, no middle ground, no gray areas. |
| **Overgeneralization** | You see a past failure or trauma as a never ending pattern of defeat or destruction. |
| **Mental Filter** | You dwell on negatives *Ex:* looking at coffee grounds and ignoring the coffee. |
| **Discounting the Positives** | You downplay accomplishments; you ignore productive possibilities of trauma. |
| **Jumping to Conclusions or Fortune Telling** | You are sure things are bad or will get worse, even though you have no proof. |
| **Mind Reading** | You are sure people are against you and thinking the worst about you. |
| **Magnification** | You blow things out of proportion, usually negative things. |
| **Minimization** | You blow off or ignore positive things, or hard issues you need to face. |
| **Emotional Reasoning** | You feel demolished and devastated now, so you decide you are ruined for life. |
| **Shoulda, Coulda, Woulda** | You criticize, and regret what should, could, would have been done or not done. |
| **Labeling** | You call yourself names or stereotype people who remind you of the enemy. |
| **Blame** | You blame yourself for events for which you were not entirely responsible, or you blame others when you have contributed to a situation. |
| **Catastrophizing** | You treat challenges as major disasters and expect the worst outcome. |
| **Excessive Self-Criticism** | You put yourself down: you are harder on yourself than you are on others. |
| **Making Demands** | You expect people to follow your orders — just as when you were in the military. |
| **Self-Fulfilling Prophecy** | You expect the worst from yourself and others, and usually get it. |
| **Personalization** | You think negative events are your fault or that things happen because of or in response to you, or to a situation you created. |

INSIGHT AND IMPOWERMENT

# Deceptions and Distortions

- Counterforce, a strategy used in nuclear warfare, targets military infrastructure.
- You can counter your cognitive distortions with positive but realistic thoughts.
- You are not expected to minimize the atrocities of war or the severity of your trauma.
- No magic cure exists to undo damage done to you and others.
- Different ways of thinking help you recover.
- Just as there are military police, you can be your own *thought police*.
- Prior examples show how your thoughts adversely affect your feelings and actions.
- The next examples and exercises show you how changing your thoughts will favorably affect your feelings and actions.

Read the negative example below; note the distortions, resultant feelings and actions.

**Thought:** *I was traumatized in combat and will never get over it.*
**Distortions:** Overgeneralization, jumping to conclusions, fortune telling.
**Feelings:** Discouragement and despair; no hope for recovery.
**Actions:** Give up on yourself; refuse help or do not seek help.

Read the positive but realistic replacement thought below; note improved feelings and actions.

**Thought:** *I was exposed to trauma, but I can get therapy and learn ways to help myself.*
**Feelings:** Awareness, acceptance, empowerment, hope.
**Actions:** Ask for treatment; join support groups; learn techniques for self-help.

## Troublesome Thoughts

**Describe your most troublesome thoughts below; identify the distortions, resultant feelings and actions. Then replace each thought, noting the improvement in feelings and actions:**

1. Negative Thought:

Distortions:

Feelings:

Actions:

**Replacement Thought:**

Feelings:

Actions:

*(Continued on the next page)*

INSIGHT AND IMPOWERMENT

# Deceptions and Distortions (continued)

**2. Negative Thought:** _____

Distortions: _____

Feelings: _____

Actions: _____

**Replacement Thought:** _____

Feelings: _____

Actions: _____

**3. Negative Thought:** _____

Distortions: _____

Feelings: _____

Actions: _____

**Replacement Thought:** _____

Feelings: _____

Actions: _____

**4. Negative Thought:** _____

Distortions: _____

Feelings: _____

Actions: _____

**Replacement Thought:** _____

Feelings: _____

Actions: _____

*(Continued on the next page)*

INSIGHT AND IMPOWERMENT

# Deceptions and Distortions (continued)

**5.** Decisive Point in military strategy is a geographic place, specific key event, critical system, or function that allows commanders to gain a marked advantage over an enemy and greatly influence the outcome of an attack.
- Your decisive point is now.
- What are the advantages of **cognitive counterforce** as illustrated by your replacement thoughts in numbers 1-4?

_____
_____
_____
_____

**6.** Consider the following quotations.
Explain why you agree or disagree with each one, and apply each one to your life:

*The basis of optimism is sheer terror.* ~ Oscar Wilde

_____
_____
_____
_____

*Oh my friend, it's not what they take away from you that counts.
It's what you do with what you have left.* ~ Hubert Humphrey

_____
_____
_____
_____

*Life is a shipwreck but we must not forget to sing in the lifeboats.* ~ Voltaire

_____
_____
_____
_____

*There is nothing either good or bad, but thinking makes it so.* ~ William Shakespeare

_____
_____
_____
_____

# Shoot and Scoot Facilitator's Guide

## Measureable Behavioral Objectives
**Veterans will ...**
- Identify, compare and contrast aspects of rational versus irrational fear.
- Describe how fear saved their lives, and how fear can sabotage them.
- State and use fear-fighting interventions.
- Utilize cognitive changes, actions, and spiritual strengths to overcome fears.
- Analyze a poem and quote, and apply those ideas to their military experience.

## Introduction
1. Before the session begins, read this guide and the reproducible pages.
2. Decide on one of the interactive variations or the traditional approach (below).
3. Photocopy reproducible pages but retain them until after the introduction.
4. Put the phrase *Shoot and Scoot* on the board and ask group members to define it in combat terms (see definition on Education and Assessment page 40).
5. Then put *Fight or Flight* on the board and discuss that these are primitive survival instincts, causing an increase in adrenaline and cortisol.
6. Encourage veterans to brainstorm the physical changes enabling fight and/or flight, such as increased heart rate and blood pressure, energized muscles, rapid breathing and blood sugar rising for fast fuel.
7. You or a volunteer lists their ideas on the board.

## Activity
1. Distribute the reproducible pages.
2. Take turns reading the Education and Assessment page aloud including the sections Rational Fear is Your Friend and Irrational Fear is Your Foe comparison.
3. Allow time to complete the written Insight and Assessment questions.
4. Encourage participants to share their answers through number 14.

## Conclusion
- Put the poem and quote on the board and read them aloud in unison, (numbers 15 and 16).
- Encourage veterans to take turns applying the poem and quote to their military experiences and their lives.

## Interactive Variations
- Ask participants to take turns reading the Insight and Empowerment questions aloud and answering orally.
- Ask them to pair up, read the questions to each other, record their partner's responses, then share with the group if they wish.

EDUCATION AND ASSESSMENT

# Shoot and Scoot

***Shoot and scoot*** is an artillery tactic to fire at a target and immediately move away from the location to avoid counter battery fire by the enemy.
- The civilian term is *fight* or *flight* (in some cases *fight and flight*).
- Fear saved you; fear can sabotage you.
- Fear mobilized you; fear can paralyze you.
- Fear of losing control or being out of control is a universal fear.
- Fear of terrorists, death and war are among the top ten fears listed in a 2005 Gallop poll.
- In combat, act first and ask questions later means heeding orders and instincts to survive.
- In civilian life, a more thoughtful response makes sense.
- Ask yourself if your current reaction relates to present danger or reverts to past experiences or events.
- FEAR = **F**alse **E**vidence or **E**xpectations **A**ppearing **R**eal

| Rational Fear is Your Friend | Irrational Fear is Your Foe |
|---|---|
| Actual danger currently exists: you are being shot at or bombed; you see death and destruction all around you. | No real danger now: you are panicked by helicopters or fireworks and/or other sights, sounds and smells that remind you of combat. |
| You must fight, flee or cover, to save your life. | You run, are ready to defend yourself, or hide out when there is no imminent threat. |
| In current combat, you act in self-defense or offense as you have been taught or ordered. | You are paralyzed by fear, or defend yourself or fight when you are not under attack. |
| The thoughts that you are in danger are valid; your life and safety are threatened. | Your thoughts about present danger are distorted, possibly flashbacks. |
| You are not ashamed of being afraid; people need strong self-preservation instincts in a war zone. | You may be embarrassed or reluctant to admit your fears as a civilian because you are not really in danger. |
| Your heart races, you feel an adrenalin rush, your muscles are energized, your senses are sharper, your rising blood sugar is fuel for battle. | You have palpitations, sweating, anxious energy, yet no external danger exists; you feel panic, the immediate physical response to irrational fear. |
| *Add your own fear* | |
| *Add your own fear* | |

INSIGHT AND EMPOWERMENT

# Shoot and Scoot

1. Describe a situation when your fear propelled you into action that kept you alive.

2. Describe a situation when you felt fear without a real threat.

3. What thoughts were you thinking before and during the episode of irrational fear?

4. Examining the evidence is a way to stay in reality. What evidence existed that proved you were not really in danger?

5. Consider this example: A veteran fears crowds and loud noises, yet his or her child plays basketball at school and desperately wants the parent at games. What was a situation wherein you or a veteran you know was actually in danger around crowds and loud noises?

6. What evidence exists that the veteran's life will not be in danger at the school's gym?

7. You may fear a panic attack in a public place like your child's game, or have other irrational fears. Using the sporting event as an example, check the boxes regarding interventions you would be willing to try.
   - ❏ Acknowledge I want to overcome fears of crowds and loud noises so I can be an involved parent and enjoy my child's sports activities.
   - ❏ Gradually desensitize myself, face my fears in baby steps, such as exposure to grocery store crowds and TV basketball games.
   - ❏ Practice relaxation techniques I can use on the spot such as deep breathing, imagining a peaceful place, repeating a phrase to myself such as "I can do this."
   - ❏ Plan an escape route: decide where I can go if I need a *time out*, such as a restroom or my car, until I feel better.
   - ❏ Take a veteran with me who has overcome similar fears; this person can coach me through my challenge.
   - ❏ Use my spiritual strengths; believe my Higher Power will protect me and empower me to do what I need to do as a parent.
   - ❏ Plan positive self talk to prevent catastrophizing, *This is merely a feeling that will pass; I am stronger each time I face my fears; the next game will be easier.*
   - ❏ Visualize myself before and during the game, enthusiastically enjoying myself.
   - ❏ Focus on how glad my child is for my support; plan how I will encourage my child whether his/her team wins or loses this game.

*(Continued on the next page)*

## INSIGHT AND EMPOWERMENT

# Shoot and Scoot *(Continued)*

8. Describe an upcoming situation or frequent source of fear for you.
   _____
   _____

9. What evidence exists to convince you the fear is unfounded?
   _____
   _____

10. What scary, irrational thoughts do you have about the situation?
    _____
    _____

11. Change the distressful thoughts to more peaceful and rational thoughts.
    _____
    _____

12. Check boxes regarding the techniques you are willing to use to prepare in advance. Feel free to add others.
    - ❑ Write about how I would behave if I did not have this fear.
    - ❑ Write about the benefits of life without this fear.
    - ❑ Talk about it to an understanding person, probably a veteran who overcame fear.
    - ❑ Seek counseling and medical care and medications if appropriate.
    - ❑ Take baby steps and gradually desensitize myself.
    - ❑ Praise myself every inch of the way.
    - ❑ Keep my eye on the prize, the positives of accomplishment.
    - ❑ _____
    - ❑ _____
    - ❑ _____

13. Check boxes for the interventions you will use during the situation. Feel free to add others.
    - ❑ Take along a buddy who has been there and done that.
    - ❑ *Fake it 'til I make it*; act as if I am brave, act my way into better thinking and feeling.
    - ❑ Feel the fear but do it anyway; just do it!
    - ❑ _____
    - ❑ _____
    - ❑ _____

14. Check boxes for the ways you will reward yourself. Feel free to add other rewards.
    - ❑ Pat myself on the back with compliments.
    - ❑ Consider how my victories are benefitting my family and other people.
    - ❑ Consider using my strengths and hopes to help other veterans struggling with fear.
    - ❑ Buy myself tangible rewards based on my budget.
    - ❑ _____
    - ❑ _____
    - ❑ _____

*(Continued on the next page)*

## INSIGHT AND EMPOWERMENT

# Shoot and Scoot *(Continued)*

15. A Poem to Consider:

### Come to the Edge

*"Come to the edge," he said.*
*They said, "We are afraid."*
*"Come to the edge," he said.*
*They came.*
*He pushed them ... and they flew.*
~ Christopher Logue

How can you push yourself to try your wings regarding something that puts you on edge?

_____
_____
_____
_____
_____
_____
_____
_____
_____
_____

16. A Quote to Consider:

*The enemy is fear. We think it is hate; but it is fear.*
~ Gandhi

Analyze and apply the Gandhi quotation to your military experience and your life.

_____
_____
_____
_____
_____
_____
_____
_____

# Swarming: Facilitator's Guide

## Measurable Behavioral Objectives
**Veterans will ...**
- Coach each other in recognizing, refuting and replacing stress-inducing thoughts.

## Introduction
1. Before the session begins, read this guide and the reproducible pages.
2. Decide on one of the interactive activities.
3. Photocopy the reproducible pages but retain them until after the introduction.
4. Write on the board the word *Swarming*, and ask its military meaning. Definition follows (#5).
5. Military *swarming* involves units of action attacking an enemy from several different directions.

## Interactive Activity Options

**Swarming** - Veterans practice attacking, refuting and replacing each other's negative thoughts:
1. Veterans sit with chairs positioned in a circle, with an empty seat in the center.
2. Distribute the reproducible *Swarming* page; each writes five disquieting thoughts.
3. Group members take turns sitting in the center chair and sharing at least one of their negative thoughts.
4. Peers take turns attacking the thought by naming its distortion, refuting or replacing it.
5. Attackers randomly shout rebuttals or replacements like bees coming from all directions.
6. A peer writes the replacements and gives them to the veteran whose thoughts were challenged.

**Pass the Paper** - Veterans practice refuting and replacing distressing thoughts in writing:
1. Participants complete the reproducible *Swarming* page, (five thoughts per person).
2. They exchange pages; everyone writes at least one replacement or rebuttal for others' thoughts.
3. Continue passing the paper until everyone has five rebuttals or replacements under each thought.
4. The papers are returned to the original owners who share a few helpful rebuttals or replacements.

**Best Buddy** - Veterans talk themselves out of negative thoughts by role-playing a conversation with a friend:
1. Veterans complete the reproducible *Swarming* page, writing five negative thoughts.
2. Pairs take turns sitting at the front of the room and exchanging papers.
3. Partner A reads one of Partner B's thoughts, pretending it is his own thought.
4. Partner B talks to Partner A as he would to a best friend, refuting and replacing (his own) thought.
5. Then they reverse roles; this continues until all participant pairs have turns.
6. Each veteran has refuted and replaced his or her own thoughts by pretending to help a best buddy.
7. Participants watching the role plays provide feedback and suggestions.

## Conclusion
- Participants state negative thoughts, then swarm their own minds with positive replacements.

INSIGHT AND EMPOWERMENT

# Swarming

**Military swarming involves units of action attacking an enemy from several different directions.**

Write five thoughts that cause you distress: anxiety, worry, fear, guilt, sadness or other emotions. Your peers will be attacking these thoughts by helping you to refute and replace them.

List your troublesome thoughts below next to each number. Leave the lines below each number blank; they will be filled in by peers later.

1. _____
   _____
   _____
   _____
   _____

2. _____
   _____
   _____
   _____
   _____

3. _____
   _____
   _____
   _____
   _____

4. _____
   _____
   _____
   _____
   _____

5. _____
   _____
   _____
   _____
   _____

# Re-Train Your Brain: Facilitator's Guide

## Measurable Behavioral Objectives
**Veterans will ...**
- Rate themselves regarding possible symptoms of Traumatic Brain Injury (TBI).
- Schedule an appointment for a medical evaluation, if needed, and document time, date, etc.
- Verbalize awareness of different types of treatment for TBI.
- Personalize the following interventions, with specifics, in writing:
    a. Substances to avoid
    b. Sleep hygiene
    c. Nutrition
    d. Gradual addition of activities alternating with rest periods
    e. Exercise for the body, mind and mood
    f. Memory, concentration, attention span improvement
    g. Better organization and loss prevention
    h. Minimize multi-tasking, distractions, interruptions
    i. Decision making precautions
    j. Patience
    k. Options for challenge and fun
    l. Cognitive change to promote recovery

## Introduction
1. Before group meets, read this guide and the reproducible pages.
2. Decide on one of the interactive variations or the traditional approach below.
3. Photocopy reproducible pages but retain them until after the introduction.
4. Write the initials *TBI* and ask if they know about this condition.
5. Ask them to share knowledge of symptoms experienced with concussions or other head injuries.
6. Explain there is much hope for recovery and a variety of treatments and self-help measures.

## Activity
1. Distribute the reproducible pages.
2. Take turns reading aloud the Education and Assessment portion.
3. Encourage participants to check the applicable boxes as they are read.
4. Allow time to complete the written Insight and Empowerment questions.
5. Encourage participants to share their responses.

## Conclusion
- Write TBI vertically and encourage them to brainstorm recovery-related words or phrases that start with each letter. Examples:

    **T:** *Think positive, Therapy helps, Treatment works, Try my best.*
    **B:** *Believe, Be all that I can be, Bravery, Bond with support group buddies.*
    **I:** *Intervene early, Insight, Inform myself, Invent a new me, Individualized treatment.*

## Interactive Variations
- Ask group members to take turns reading the Insight and Empowerment questions aloud and answering orally.
- Ask group members to pair up with peers, read the questions to each other, record their partner's responses, then share with the group if they wish.

EDUCATION AND ASSESSMENT

# Re-Train Your Brain

**TBI** — Traumatic Brain Injury ranges from mild (like a concussion) to severe brain injuries. It can be caused by bullets, blasts, falls, vehicular crashes, assaults, fragments such as shrapnel, etc.

An injury to the head may result in many of the symptoms below.
**Check the boxes of those that apply to you:**
- ❑ Suffered a head injury, exposed to explosions in combat
- ❑ Dazed or lost consciousness after the injury
- ❑ Frequent headaches
- ❑ Neck pain
- ❑ Problems with dizziness, poor balance
- ❑ Memory, learning, attention span, retention or concentration difficulties
- ❑ Problem–solving and decision-making difficulties; easily distracted
- ❑ Too much or too little sleep; restlessness
- ❑ Extreme fatigue, little motivation
- ❑ Ringing in the ears
- ❑ Change in sex drive
- ❑ Easily irritated, angry with little provocation
- ❑ Slow thinking, acting, speaking, reading; confusion
- ❑ Problems with task organization
- ❑ Sensitivity to sounds, lights, distractions; blurred vision, loss of the sense of smell
- ❑ Moody, sad or anxious
- ❑ Bowel or bladder control problems

Because there are many possible reasons for some of the above symptoms, and early intervention helps recovery, you must see your local Veteran's Administration physician or your primary care MD. Additionally any of the following may be recommended:

- Occupational therapy to help you with activities of daily living
- Physical therapy to help you walk, exercise, and use assistive devices
- Speech therapy if your language skills are impaired
- Psychological therapy to help you cope emotionally
- Psychiatry if there are co-occurring PTS(D) or mood disorders that need medications
- Social work or case management if you need referrals to resources to coordinate your care
- Therapies to improve thinking, learning, concentration, problem-solving and decision-making
- Art therapy to help you express feelings and thoughts non-verbally
- Recreational therapy, enjoyable activities that help concentration, memory, and organization
- Driver rehabilitation to re-learn or improve driving skills
- Vocational rehabilitation to help with school, training, and employment
- Vestibular therapy to help you restore your equilibrium and balance
- Neurology consult

INSIGHT AND EMPOWERMENT

# Re-Train Your Brain

1. **If you have not been evaluated for Traumatic Brain Injury and have symptoms**, make note of the date, time and location of your appointment

   a. **Date** _____  **Time** _____  **Location** _____

2. **The Care and Feeding of Your Brain**

   a. **Don't slow it down:** Avoid alcohol and sleep aids that slow down your thinking, memory and recovery and increase re-injury risks. If you use them, state how you plan to stop:

   _____
   _____
   _____
   _____

   b. **Don't rev it up:** Avoid caffeine, energy products and ephedrine in over the counter cold remedies. These increase anxiety and irritability. If you use products like these, state how you plan to stop:

   _____
   _____
   _____
   _____

   c. **If you don't snooze you lose:** Without sleeping pills, promote 7 to 9 hours sleep by avoiding stimulants; getting plenty of exercise early in the day; sticking to a wake-sleep schedule; taking minimal short naps; keeping bedroom cool and dark, with no noise or a noise that blocks out sounds or relaxes you; using imagery, breathing deeply, meditation, prayer, progressive muscle relaxation and other techniques. You may ask your doctor about herbal supplements, but do not use these without medical advice.

   _____
   _____
   _____
   _____

   d. **Feed your Brain:** Recommendations emphasize whole grains; colorful vegetables; fruits versus juices; fish, nuts, healthy vegetable oils; no fat or low fat foods; lean meat, poultry, fish, eggs and legumes. Describe a daily meal plan for yourself:

   _____
   _____
   _____
   _____
   _____

*(Continued on the next page)*

## INSIGHT AND EMPOWERMENT

# Re-Train Your Brain *(Continued)*

3. **Retrain Your Brain**

   a. **Don't overdo or under-do:** Jumping into the swing of everything may overwhelm you; staying on the sidelines too long may foster fear and reluctance to re-emerge. Fatigue may make you more irritable. How will you balance periods of activity with rest?
   _____
   _____

   b. **Jog your mind:** Exercise helps body, mind and mood. Do what you enjoy earlier in the day, not too close to bedtime. Write a schedule of types of exercise you will do each week and when:
   _____
   _____

   c. **Jog your memory:** Keep a notepad in your pocket or purse or carry a notebook; write what you need to remember; refer to it often! What kinds of information do you need to keep at your fingertips?
   _____
   _____

   d. **Organize yourself:** Have a written Things to Do list and cross off accomplishments. Prioritize tasks, but re-adjust priorities as needed. Some things will slide over into tomorrow, and that's ok. Begin your list now on the reverse side of this page or a blank sheet.
   _____
   _____

   e. **A place for everything and everything in its place:** losing items may be part of TBI; practice putting things in the same place. What items do you often lose and where can you keep them?
   _____
   _____

   f. **Avoid multi-tasking:** Do one thing at time, try to minimize distractions and interruptions. What are important tasks to complete and how can you cut down distractions and interruptions?
   _____
   _____

   g. **Delay decisions:** you may be a bit impulsive; talk with a trusted person; think things through; practice problem-solving skills. What current or upcoming decisions will you need to address?
   _____
   _____

   h. **The waiting game:** many brain injuries are resolved fairly quickly, but some take longer. Have patience with yourself; focus on your strides; cheer yourself on. What improvements have you already seen in yourself?
   _____
   _____

   i. **Mind-games:** Some people increase their memory, concentration and attention span by playing board games, cards, and doing crossword and other puzzles; others are easily frustrated and quickly feel defeated. What types of challenges will you try? When will you schedule them during each day or week?
   _____
   _____

   j. **Thoughts, Feelings & Actions:** A positive attitude facilitates recovery. Write a self-defeating thought that holds you back; then write a positive but realistic replacement and note how your emotions and actions will change:
   _____
   _____

# Anger

*"Anger is a great force. If you can control it, it can be transmuted into a power which can move the whole world."*

~ William Shenstone

Post-deployment anger and underlying fears and needs are common amongst veterans. In this chapter, veterans have the opportunity to identify reasons for these emotions and learn to calm themselves and others by practicing conflict resolution and to replace anger inducing distortions with anger-reducing thoughts. The participants will address risks for domestic violence and safety issues.

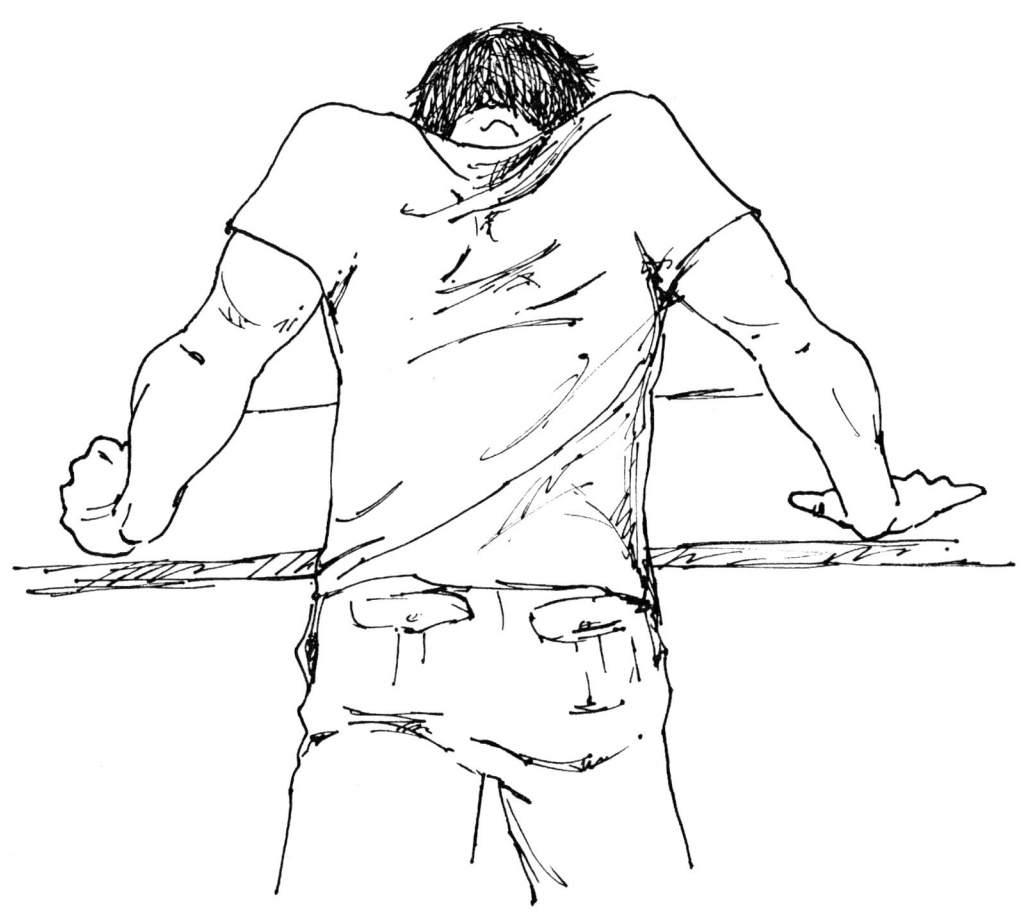

# Anguish and Anger Facilitator's Guide

## Measurable Behavioral Objectives
**Veterans will ...**
- Identify factors related to the disruption in their lives due to deployment and the suffering from war that might lead to anger.
- Identify conditions that may pre-dispose them to anger problems.
- Identify universal fears underlying most anger.
- Express their anger orally and/or in writing or by drawing.
- Decide on quick ways to decrease anger.
- Identify stumbling blocks to resolving anger issues.
- Acknowledge ways to change their outlook and outcomes.
- Apply quotations to their lives regarding military-related or personal anger issues.

## Introduction
1. Before the session begins, read this guide and the reproducible pages.
2. Decide on one of the interactive variations or the traditional approach (below). Photocopy the reproducible pages but retain them until after the introduction.
3. Ask participants to brainstorm reasons for veterans to feel anger.
4. You or a volunteer participant lists their responses on the board. Validate feelings.
5. Ask group members to brainstorm possible consequences of acting aggressively and list them on the board.
6. Explain that they will be helped to deal with reactions to their disrupted lives and suffering.

## Activity
1. Distribute the reproducible pages and ask veterans to take turns reading aloud the Education and Assessment portion.
2. Encourage the group members to check the applicable boxes as they are read.
3. Allow time to complete the written Insight and Empowerment questions.
4. Encourage participants to share their responses through Number 10.

## Conclusion
- Encourage participants to share their responses to the quotation, Number 11.

## Interactive Variations
- Ask participants to read aloud the Insight and Empowerment questions and answer them orally.
- Ask them to pair up with peers, read the questions to each other, record their partner's responses, and then share with the group if they wish.

## Teams
1. People indicate whether they usually tend to be passive or aggressive and divide into two teams.
2. Each team goes to a separate side of the room and elects a recorder to list their ideas.
3. Passive people brainstorm how to be more direct and open.
4. Aggressive people brainstorm ways to be assertive.
5. The groups re-unite and their recorders share their lists, eliciting input from the other team.
6. Recorders add input from the other team.
7. The lists are photocopied and distributed to all participants.

EDUCATION AND ASSESSMENT

# Anguish and Anger

Anger may be justifiable, especially after combat exposure and/or being away from familiar surroundings, and friends and family. Environmental conditions such as deserts, extreme temperatures or terrains, foreign cultures, distasteful food probably irritated you; death and destruction may have enraged you.

**Passive or passive aggressive responses; check those that apply to you:**

- ❏ Stuffing anger by not talking about it; acting untouched; smiling when I feel like screaming.
- ❏ Using substances or meaningless sex to escape feelings.
- ❏ Becoming obsessed with games, computers or other diversions.
- ❏ Evading and avoiding conflicts or crises.
- ❏ Giving half-hearted effort toward resolution.
- ❏ Going to extremes in other areas of life such as cleanliness, over or under-eating, checking and re-checking excessively.
- ❏ Stockpiling resentments.
- ❏ Blaming self too much or being too self-sacrificing.
- ❏ Complaining behind people's backs.
- ❏ Disobeying rules.
- ❏ Exaggerating illness or injury to make others feel guilty or to get my own way.

**Aggressive expressions of anger; check those that apply to you:**

- ❏ Bullying physically or verbally.
- ❏ Road rage.
- ❏ Damaging people verbally or physically.
- ❏ Property destruction; breaking objects.
- ❏ Harming animals.
- ❏ Expecting *center stage*, talking above others, showing off, especially with reckless behavior.
- ❏ Intimidating others with physical prowess, power or rank.
- ❏ Threatening, stigmatizing or blaming people or groups.
- ❏ Unpredictable and explosive behavior; raging.
- ❏ Holding grudges, refusing to make-up or forgive, not accepting apologies or apologizing.
- ❏ Unfair fighting such as bringing up the past or *hitting below the belt*.
- ❏ Scapegoating.
- ❏ Displacing fury onto weaker, probably blameless victims.

INSIGHT AND EMPOWERMENT

# Anguish and Anger

1. **Deployment, a disruption in your life, and suffering from war can easily lead to anger. Check the boxes that apply to you:**
   - ❏ I left school for the military.
   - ❏ I left my job for the military.
   - ❏ My career was set back as colleagues moved ahead.
   - ❏ I lost my job.
   - ❏ My income decreased.
   - ❏ My family cohesion suffered from being geographically distant.
   - ❏ My partner and I and/or my family are now emotionally distant.
   - ❏ My friends and I have drifted apart.
   - ❏ I resent the war because I suffered stress, sadness and/or losses.
   - ❏ I am angry at officials regarding their decisions.
   - ❏ I am angry about delays in getting benefits and help.
   - ❏ I was forced to do things against my conscience or morals.
   - ❏ I lost my position of power within my family.
   - ❏ I have physical and/or emotional injuries.
   - ❏ Civilians do not understand what I went through.
   - ❏ I think I was not sufficiently trained for combat, the region, or nuclear or chemical attack.
   - ❏ I feel my sacrifices are unappreciated.
   - ❏ I think I was not appropriately debriefed after trauma.
   - ❏ I underwent sexual, gender or sexual identity harassment or abuse.
   - ❏ I am constantly on alert, fearing attack.
   - ❏ I have poor concentration and sleep patterns.
   - ❏ I have symptoms of PTSD, especially the hyper-vigilance noted above.
   - ❏ I have symptoms of TBI, traumatic brain injury.
   - ❏ I fired a weapon during deployment.
   - ❏ I served lengthy or multiple deployments.
   - ❏ I was exposed to combat.
   - ❏ I deployed at a young age.

2. **Other factors may pre-dispose you to anger. Check the boxes that apply to you:**
   - ❏ I was physically or sexually abused in childhood.
   - ❏ I witnessed family violence in childhood.
   - ❏ I was overly controlled by others or treated as insignificant in childhood.
   - ❏ I have been exploited by others.
   - ❏ I was verbally abused with frequent put-downs in childhood.
   - ❏ I received no nurturing, understanding, guidance, protection in childhood.
   - ❏ I have been placed in vulnerable situations, helpless to defend myself from abuse.
   - ❏ I use illegal substances, alcohol or prescription drugs.

3. **It has been said that three fears underlie anger. Check the boxes that apply to you:**
   - ❏ **Fear of abandonment:** I fear that I am and/or will be alone; I fear lack of emotional support from my partner, family, friends or community.
   - ❏ **Fear loss of self-esteem:** I fear being perceived as weak if I suffer symptoms or need help.
   - ❏ **Fear of loss of control over a situation:** I had little control over combat and war strategy decisions; I fear inability to resume control over my life, and my emotions and recovery.

*(Continued on the next page)*

## INSIGHT AND EMPOWERMENT

# Anguish and Anger *(continued)*

**4. What other factors explain your anger issues?**
_____
_____


**5. Some people are helped by talking to a trusted person, a good listener, who will not interrupt or cut you off. Other people's anger intensifies when they express it. You may be able to express your anger via drawing, painting, poetry, journaling or music.**

What person will you talk to? _____

When? _____

**6. If you cannot speak with a helpful person soon, perhaps writing about your anger, the situations and your responses, might help.**

Who was involved? _____

What happened? _____

Where? _____

When? _____

Why did it happen? _____

Why did it anger you? _____

How did you handle the people, situation and your feelings? _____
_____
_____
_____

**7. Constructive versus destructive anger is discussed below. Check items with which you agree:**

❏ Anger is a normal response and can be helpful in self-preservation and in correcting injustices.

❏ Crying is cathartic, not wimpy.

❏ Constructive anger is acknowledged, does not have detrimental consequences, and can be worked out to meet my own and others' needs.

❏ Destructive anger has consequences such as hurting others, legal charges, remorse; it usually simmers and turns inward into depression or self-harm, or erupts into violence or verbal aggression.

*(Continued on the next page)*

## INSIGHT AND EMPOWERMENT

# Anguish and Anger *(continued)*

8. **Some quick ways to deal with anger are listed below. Check the methods you have used or will try:**
   ❑ Talk-it-out or write-it-out.
   ❑ Work-it-out: exercise to release pent-up peeves.
   ❑ Time-out from the situation and/or person(s).
   ❑ Chill-out: sooth myself with music, art, journaling, nature, spirituality.
   ❑ Zone-out with distractions, movies, books, tasks, enjoyable activities.
   ❑ Relax with deep breathing and/or progressive muscle relaxation.
   ❑ Guided imagery tapes or my own imagery or visualization.
   ❑ Conflict resolution skills.

9. **Be aware of the stumbling blocks. Check the boxes that apply to you:**
   ❑ I deny or minimize the severity of my anger.
   ❑ I blame others or situations outside of myself.
   ❑ I believe I was wronged but do not look at MY role in the problem.
   ❑ I express my anger too loudly and too intensely, and then it becomes worse.
   ❑ I make others give in to me because of my aggression, and this results in relationship problems.
   ❑ I have rigid rules for others and I am angry when people are not perfect.
   ❑ I am angry with myself if I fall short of my own standards.
   ❑ I am angry when situations and outcomes do not suit my demands.

10. **Changing your outlook may change your outcomes. Check the techniques you use or will consider:**
    ❑ Admit I overreact regarding anger.
    ❑ Recognize I cannot control people or circumstances.
    ❑ Realize I am in control of my own reactions.
    ❑ Know when expressing anger will help.
    ❑ Awareness of when expressing my feelings will exasperate me or escalate the other person's anger.
    ❑ Recognize that compromise is better for a relationship than intimidating people to comply with my every wish.
    ❑ Stop expecting others to obey my rules, unless they are my children or subordinates; then cut some slack for their human imperfections.
    ❑ Be gentler with myself.
    ❑ Remind myself that, unfortunately, situations happen.
    ❑ Decide I can dislike a circumstance or a person's behavior without becoming enraged.
    ❑ Recognize that people have free choice and will not often do things on purpose to please or displease me; they have their own motivations; I do not need to take their behavior personally.
    ❑ Remember that taking revenge hurts me and forgiveness helps me.

*(Continued on the next page)*

INSIGHT AND EMPOWERMENT

# Anguish and Anger (continued)

11. Many minds have pondered anger. Read the quotations and apply them to your military or personal experiences:

    *Anger is a killing thing: it kills the man who angers, for each rage leaves him less than he was before – it takes something from him.* ~ Louis L'Amour

    *Get mad, then get over it.* ~ Colin Powell

    *When anger rises, think of the consequences.* ~ Confucius

    *He who angers you conquers you.* ~ Elizabeth Kenny

    *The world needs anger. The world often continues to allow evil because it isn't angry enough.* ~ Bede Jarrett

    *Always forgive your enemies – nothing annoys them so much.* ~ Oscar Wilde

    *Always write angry letters to your enemies. Never mail them.* ~ James Fallows

    *Anger is an acid that can do more harm to the vessel in which it is stored than to anything on which it is poured.* ~ Mark Twain

    *Anger, if not restrained, is frequently more hurtful to us than the injury that provokes it.*
    ~ Lucius Annaeus Seneca

    *There are two things a person should never be angry at, what they can help, and what they cannot.* ~ Plato

# De-Escalation: Learn the Language Facilitator's Guide

## Measurable Behavioral Objectives
**Veterans will ...**
- State stages of the Escalation Cycle and acknowledge the value of early intervention.
- Acknowledge aspects of de-escalation for potentially dangerous anger.
- Practice interventions for non-violent anger situations.
- Practice steps in conflict resolution.
- Describe an unfulfilled need at the root of their anger.

## Introduction
1. Before the session begins, read this guide and the reproducible pages.
2. Decide on one of the interactive variations or the traditional approach (below).
3. Photocopy the reproducible pages but retain them until after the introduction.
4. Before group enlist two volunteers to pantomime a sketch; let them practice out of sight of the group.
5. One acts angry, clenching fists, stomping feet, mumbling under his or her breath.
6. The other turns away, folds arms across chest in an uninterested manner, rolls eyes, and then faces the person, stands up, puts hands on hips and shakes index finger at the angry one.
7. After practicing, the two *players* perform for the *audience*.
8. People clap and the *performers* take their seats.
9. Ask the *actors* and group to discuss what the skit portrayed, eliciting that there was an angry person and the partner was refusing to listen, then seemed to give orders or reprimand, all via body language.

## Activity
1. Distribute the reproducible pages.
2. Take turns reading the Education and Assessment portion aloud.
3. Allow time to complete the written Insight and Empowerment questions.
4. Encourage participants to share their responses through number 9.

## Conclusion
- Encourage participants to share their responses to the quotation (number 10).

## Interactive Variations
- Ask participants to take turns reading the Insight and Empowerment questions aloud and answering orally.
- Ask participants to pair up with peers, read the questions to each other, record their partner's responses, then share with the group if they wish.

**Role-Play**
1. Two volunteers sit in the front of the room or center of the circle.
2. A third volunteer plays the coach and sits by.
3. The two volunteers have previously decided on a conflict to portray.
4. The two role play their conflict.
5. The coach prompts them to use each step.
6. Peers assist with brainstorming if they have additional ideas after step number 7.
7. At the end of each practice session, peers provide feedback regarding how the volunteers handled the conflict.

EDUCATION AND ASSESSMENT

# De-Escalation: Learn the Language

You have probably experienced your own anger and other people's wrath. Learning how to calm people down and resolve conflicts will help you and others deal with the issues arising from your military experience, changing roles and other issues.

## The Escalation Cycle involves five stages:

1. **Activation:** an external event such as delays in getting benefits or an internal event such as a flashback or anxiety attack.
2. **Escalation:** anger simmers and intensifies; physical manifestations may include clenched jaw and fists, red face, mumbling, swearing; alternately some people become quiet and withdrawn.
3. **Crisis:** threats, actions such as punching walls or people.
4. **De-escalation:** energy is discharged during crisis; the person's rage is calming down.
5. **Recovery:** following de-escalation, usually the person is apologetic and remorseful and may sleep from exhaustion.

**Early Intervention is the Key** — The earlier you intervene and implement the active listening and empathy steps suggested below, the less likely the person is to go into full blown crisis.

## De-Escalation Action Plan

1. **Think safety first.**
2. **If necessary, leave the situation** and/or call 911 or your Emergency Services number.
3. **If you decide it is safe to use de-escalation tactics, implement these steps:**

- **Pay attention** by muting the TV or music, putting down your book, stopping your task.
- **Use open body language** by facing the person, standing or sitting with arms open, not crossed or on your hips.
- **Control facial expressions** including no frowns or rolling your eyes.
- **Listen** and let the person vent; do not try to defend yourself or make the person see the situation differently; at this time the person has *tunnel vision*.
- **Feel the person's pain** by responding to the emotional content, not the facts of the situation.
- **Ask how**, not why. You are neither detective nor judge; you are not trying to sort out facts, and questions such as *Why?* puts them on the defensive; ask how things started, how did they feel, what happened, etc.
- **Prove you get it** by paraphrasing or repeating in your own words the gist of the situation and their response, *I'd feel ignored and insulted too if I were treated that way; I can understand how you feel disrespected when I do that.*
- **Contribute to calmness** but do not say, *Calm down:* the person would have calmed down if he/she could; as the person realizes your understanding, it will de-escalate the anger.
- **Suggest soothing techniques** such as, *Are you able to try some deep breathing? Would you like to sit down and have a (non-alcoholic) drink or snack? Do you want to just be left alone?*
- **Short term tactics** such as, *Let's consider getting help from a counselor, (or attorney if the person's issue entails legalities); A little later, let's both think about ways we can help the situation.*

EDUCATION AND ASSESSMENT

# De-Escalation

## After averting a crisis, or in non-violent situations, consider these interventions

1. **Tact:** use the kindest, most tactful terms possible versus hiding or stuffing your feelings, or attacking.
2. **Empathy:** see the situation from the other person's point of view; feel the person's emotions versus your side only.
3. **Respect:** respect the person's right to see things his/her own way versus insisting he/she agrees. Do not demean or belittle the person.
4. **Resolution:** try to resolve issues rather than you or the other person remaining resentful, a victim, or stubbornly refusing to budge.
5. **Education:** learn versus keeping a closed mind.
6. **Let go:** decide it's over versus fanning the flame, or even getting a *high* from your personal fury.
7. **Self-Examination:** look at your role in the conflict versus totally blaming the person.
8. **Validity:** believe the person has valid thoughts and feelings which may be different from your views.
9. **Commitment:** decide the person and relationship are more important than the issue at hand.
10. **Win-Win:** decide to compromise versus insisting there must be a winner and a loser.

## Conflict Resolution Skills

**Helpful steps when both parties are calm enough and willing to work together:**

1. **Clear the air:** if you are disgruntled or the person is agitated, say *it seems like we need to talk ...*
2. **Time out:** suggest a brief break; agree on a time to discuss issues; *can we talk in half an hour?*
3. **Ground Rules:** agree to stick to the issue; not bring up the past; no threats or violence; mutual respect.
4. **Active listening:** be quiet; be sure you hear the person's perspective.
5. **Summarize the person's views and feelings:** prove you understand by restating concerns.
6. **Ask permission to talk about your thoughts and feelings:** then do not attack; use I-messages - say *I feel hurt when that happens;* do not say *you always...you never...you make me feel...*
7. **Brainstorm with pen and paper:** encourage outrageous ideas; laugh; workable solutions may emerge.
8. **Agree on plausible possibilities:** cross off options neither of you want; keep the ones you like.
9. **Pros and Cons:** list the advantages and disadvantages of each idea; agree, or try *Plan A*, then *Plan B*.
10. **Compromise:** agree on a fifty-fifty split, or a forty-sixty compromise; seek a win-win outcome.

**In the event of the worst-case-scenario, consider these thoughts and actions:**

1. You care about the person but he/she is truly being unreasonable.
2. You have tried all of the above techniques but serious issues remain.
3. Consider counseling for both of you to maintain your peace of mind and to protect yourself and family. Decide together how to handle the situation.
4. You go for counseling alone, if necessary.
5. Attempt to convince the other person to also seek counseling.
6. You can decide to react appropriately, no matter what, versus stooping to a level of cruelty or combativeness you will eventually regret.

INSIGHT AND EMPOWERMENT

# De-Escalation

1. Consider a recent heated exchange with a person you care about. Share how you responded:

2. Write a tactful statement you need to say to this person regarding a current behavior or situation.
   *Example:* **instead of** *you are clueless about my suffering* **say** *it is hard for people who were not there to understand the effects of combat or how combat affected me.*

3. Write a statement showing you understand this person's emotions regarding a current situation:

4. Give an example of a time you held resentment or refused to compromise on an issue:

5. Tell about a time you actually were energized in a negative way by your anger and fueled by your self-righteous indignation:

6. What were the results of hanging on versus letting go of your wrath?

7. What is your role in a recent or current conflict?

8. What are some valid points the other person has stated?

9. Explain whether and how the person and relationship are more important than the issue at hand:

10. Apply this quote to your anger and state a better way to meet your need:

    *At the core of all anger is a need that is not being fulfilled.* ~ Marshall B. Rosenberg

# Inducing or Reducing Anger? Facilitator's Guide

## Measurable Behavioral Objectives

Veterans will ...

- Reframe anger inducing and distorted thoughts to anger-reducing thoughts.

## Introduction

1. Before the session begins, read this guide and the reproducible pages.
2. Decide on one of the interactive variations or the traditional approach (below).
3. Photocopy the reproducible pages, but retain them until after the introduction.
4. Write on the board: *Why are many veterans angry?*
5. Encourage brainstorming and list participants' reasons on the board.
6. Explain that how we think can induce or reduce our anger.

## Activity

1. Distribute the reproducible pages.
2. Take turns reading the Education and Assessment portion aloud.
3. Allow time to complete the written Insight and Empowerment questions.
4. Encourage participants to share their responses.

## Conclusion

- Encourage participants to share a time their attitude made them more or less angry.

## Interactive Variations

- Ask participants to take turns reading each Insight and Empowerment example aloud and sharing their responses orally.
- Ask individuals to pair up with peers, read the distortions to each other, record the partner's responses, then share with the group if they wish.

EDUCATION AND ASSESSMENT & INSIGHT AND EMPOWERMENT

# Inducing or Reducing Anger?

## Education and Assessment

**Please Note:**
Obtain professional help for severe anger issues. If your rage endangers yourself or others, call 911 or your local Emergency Services number, the National Suicide Prevention Lifeline/Veteran's Crisis Line, 1-800-273-8255 (TALK), or go to your nearest hospital Emergency Room.

- How you think can affect whether you are aggressive or assertive, resentful or forgiving.
- Your thoughts can inflame you or cool you down.
- Consider that the person you are mad at is usually a loved one, and that you do value the relationship.
- You can hope people's behavior will improve, but you can also alter your attitude toward them.
- If your anger is at the military, there are channels for communication and change.
- You cannot change the past; you can change your reactions so you are not destroyed by anger.

## Insight and Empowerment

Consider the following examples, and practice changing your thoughts:

**All or Nothing, no middle ground:** *He thinks he is a hero because he handled home responsibilities.*
Re-think: *We are both important; let's recognize each other's contributions.*
All or Nothing: _____
Re-think: _____

**Mental Filter, focus only on negatives:** *I'm so angry about the atrocities of war; what I saw and had to do.*
Re-think: *Combat was terrible but I developed some personal strengths.*
Mental Filter: _____
Re-think: _____

**Fortune Telling, assuming outcomes:** *They put me through so much misery; I'll never recover.*
Re-think: *I endured a lot and have changed; I will eventually move forward.*
Fortune Telling: _____
Re-think: _____

**Mind Reading, believing you know what people think:** *My partner thinks I'm stupid, a doormat, etc.*
Re-think: *I will ask what my partner thinks instead of assuming; I need to know the truth about myself.*
Mind Reading: _____
Re-think: _____

**Emotional Reasoning, anger overrides your brain:** *I'm so angry about delays I'll cancel my appointment.*
Re-think: *I don't like waiting, but I am doing what I can to help myself in the meantime.*
Emotional Reasoning: _____
Re-think: _____

**Shoulds, trying to dictate people's behavior:** *She should show more consideration for my feelings.*
Re-think: *She is involved in her own issues; I'll share more about my feelings and hope she listens.*
Shoulds: _____
Re-think: _____

INSIGHT AND EMPOWERMENT

# Inducing or Reducing Anger? *(Continued)*

**Blaming, trying to see who is at fault versus solving a problem or resolving an issue:** *It's his fault I feel miserable.*
Re-think: *My attitude toward this difficulty is my responsibility.*
Blaming: _____
Re-think: _____

**Catastrophizing, expecting disaster:** *These employers think I have no skills; I'll never get hired.*
Re-think: *I'll explain my transferrable skills or get training; I'll check into companies that hire veterans.*
Catastrophizing: _____
Re-think: _____

**Excessive Self-Criticism, put downs:** *I'm a terrible partner; we argue because of me.*
Re-think: *I take responsibility for my role, but two are in this relationship.*
Excessive Self-Criticism: _____
Re-think: _____

**Making Demands or threats:** *They will give me my benefits now or I'll give them a piece of my mind.*
Re-think: *I'll make my needs known; I'll ask to speak with a supervisor; I'll use the chain of command.*
Making Demands: _____
Re-think: _____

**Personalization, self-blame:** *I'm angry at myself for what I did in combat; people got hurt or died because of me.*
Re-think: *I did the best I could at the time; things happen in combat that are no one's fault.*
Personalization: _____
Re-think: _____

**Self Fulfilling Prophesy, you get what you expect:** *I'm doomed because of the military's decisions.*
Re-think: *I can empower myself to use the resources available and develop coping skills.*
Self Fulfilling Prophesy: _____
Re-think: _____

**Overgeneralization, stereotypes:** *Civilians are clueless about the horror I have been through.*
Re-think: *I will share information, within my comfort level and some might understand.*
Overgeneralization: _____
Re-think: _____

**Labeling, self or others:** *I'm a time bomb waiting to explode; he's an idiot.*
Re-think: *I need help with anger management; how he thinks is his own business, not mine.*
Labeling: _____
Re-think: _____

# Risks for Domestic Violence Facilitator's Guide

## Measurable Behavioral Objectives

**Veterans will ...**
- Rate relationships regarding risks specific to military couples.
- Identify characteristics of abusers.
- Rate themselves or partner regarding types of emotional abuse.
- Rate themselves or partner regarding types of physical abuse.
- Read *The Abuse Cycle* aloud and apply it to their situation.
- Describe their feelings regarding their role in aspects of the cycle.
- Take steps to break the abuse cycle or prevent it by seeking professional assistance if needed.

## Introduction

1. Before group meets, read this guide and the reproducible pages.
2. Decide on one of the interactive activities or the traditional approach (below).
3. Photocopy the reproducible pages but retain them until after the introduction.
4. Put a circle on the board. Title it *The Abuse Cycle*.
5. Label as follows clockwise: around the 2 o'clock, Tension Building; around the 4 o'clock,
6. Incident; around 8 o'clock, Reconciliation; around 10:00, Calm.
7. Ask group members to discuss aspects of each phase, based on their labels.
8. Explain that they will be addressing special risks for military couples.

## Activity

1. Distribute the reproducible pages.
2. Take turns reading the Education and Assessment pages aloud.
3. Encourage group members to check the applicable boxes as they are read.
4. Allow time to complete the written Insight and Empowerment questions.
5. Encourage group members to share their answers through number 3.

## Conclusion

- Encourage group members to share their insights, number 4.

## Interactive Variations

- Ask participants to take turns reading the Insight and Empowerment questions aloud and answering orally.
- Ask participants to pair up with peers, read the questions to each other, record their partner's responses, then share with the group if they wish.

EDUCATION AND ASSESSMENT

# Risks for Domestic Violence

Military couples are at risk for emotional, physical, sexual, verbal, and financial abuse. Domestic violence occurs in all racial, ethnic, age, cultural, educational, and socio-economic groups, and in all military ranks.

**Check factors that apply to your relationship:**
- ❑ Frequent deployments and reintegration
- ❑ Frequent re-location, away from friends, family, support systems
- ❑ Economic dependence among many military spouses or partners
- ❑ Living off-base outside of the United States

**Check boxes of characteristics of abusers that apply to you or to your partner:**
- ❑ Abuse of alcohol or drugs
- ❑ Abuse witnessed in childhood
- ❑ Victim of abuse as a child
- ❑ Abuse of or by prior partners
- ❑ Abuse of pets
- ❑ Unemployment or underemployment
- ❑ Control of partner's activities
- ❑ Control of money and partner's access to funds
- ❑ Control of partner's contact with family and friends
- ❑ Harmful threats toward partner or children
- ❑ Revenge regarding custody; false allegations of child abuse
- ❑ Suicide threats if partner tries to separate
- ❑ Sabotage partner's work or school efforts
- ❑ Unpredictability of moods with anger outbursts
- ❑ Untreated emotional conditions

**Emotional abuse is serious. Check boxes that apply to you or your partner:**
- ❑ Put-downs, name calling, words to make partner feel worthless and stupid
- ❑ Jealously, insistence partner is cheating
- ❑ Punishment of partner by silent treatment and withholding affection
- ❑ Criticism of partner's children
- ❑ Angry about an unplanned pregnancy
- ❑ Blame placed on partner for arguments and problems
- ❑ Refusal to let partner sleep at night
- ❑ Threats to reveal embarrassing secrets if partner tries to leave
- ❑ Use of threatening or intimidating body language or verbal threats

**Physical abuse is serious. Check those that apply to you or your partner:**
- ❑ Destroying property during an argument
- ❑ Pushing, slapping, punching, biting, hair pulling, shoving, choking, kicking, etc.
- ❑ Threatening with a weapon
- ❑ Driving recklessly with partner or children in the car
- ❑ Forcing sex or pressuring partner to do acts against their will
- ❑ Keeping the partner and/or children hostage in the residence
- ❑ Preventing partner from calling police or reporting abuse
- ❑ Withholding medication

EDUCATION AND ASSESSMENT *(Continued)* & INSIGHT AND EMPOWERMENT

# The Abuse Cycle

**Most experts agree a series of events replay. Below is a summary of The Abuse Cycle:**
**Tension Building:** the victim tries to avoid triggering an outburst.
**Acute Battering Episode:** acting-out phase, violent incident; abuser dominates.
**Honeymoon or Incident Reconciliation:** affection and apology by the abuser.
**Calm Phase:** temporary peace before the inevitable recurring storm of tension building.

## Alert

If you are an abuser or a potential abuser, get professional help before irreparable damage is done.
If you feel victimized, do not build up resentment and then react violently. Turning the tables backfires.
Seek safety and survive. In a domestic violence situation, call 911 or your local Emergency Services number, or leave the situation and go to a place of safety immediately. Do not drive if you are enraged.

**Consider the following:**
- Think Safety First. Leave a volatile situation while you and partner have life and limb intact.
- You can always reconsider reconciliation, later, after you and your partner receive help.
- Remember, hope and healing are available. Ask!
- Get help for yourselves and for the children's safety and emotional health.
- Ideally both partners can access the services suggested in this activity and in the Resources chapter, pages 159–163.
- Abusers can learn anger management and develop insight.
- Survivors can improve self-esteem and assertive skills.
- Treatment exists for substance abuse and mental health issues which often contribute to violence.

## Insight and Empowerment

Describe your feelings regarding these statements:

1. How does the Abuse Cycle usually play out in your situation?

2. Unequal power – In what ways are you too powerful or powerless?

3. Humiliation – In what ways are you degrading your partner or children, or being put–down by your partner?

4. Isolation – In what ways do you cut off your partner's support system or are you restricted from your support system?

5. Intimidation – In what ways are you frightening your partner or children, or being terrorized by your partner?

6. Blame – In what ways are you pointing the finger or being the target of blame?

7. Guilt – In what ways are you feeling remorse for abusing your partner or children, or for blaming yourself for your partner's aggression?

8. Denial – In what ways are you playing down your violence toward your partner or children, or having your pain minimized?

9. Set-up – In what ways are you craving and creating fights with your partner or children, or walking on eggshells to avoid battles?

INSIGHT AND EMPOWERMENT

# Breaking the Abuse Cycle

1. Talk with a therapist, counselor, spiritual or religious leader, family member or friend. Whom will you contact?
   _____

2. Talk to your partner and ask him/her to go with you for couples counseling. The local Veteran's Administration, or your health insurance's Behavioral Health benefits can refer you to marital-couples counseling.

   When and how will you approach your partner?
   _____
   _____
   _____
   _____
   _____

3. Websites for Military Home Front and Military One Source explain about the Family Advocacy Program (FAP), which provides assessment, education and treatment. Family Support Centers provide education, referral, and help with couples issues including anger and stress management, parenting, etc. Check http://www.ndvh for the National Domestic Violence Hotline. They provide numbers for inside and outside the U.S., and for people with hearing impairments.

   What is the time and date for your appointment or referral from Family Advocacy, Family Support, your insurance company's referral or your County Mental Health services or other resource?
   _____
   _____
   _____
   _____
   _____

4. Summarize the most valuable insights developed today:
   _____
   _____
   _____
   _____
   _____
   _____
   _____
   _____
   _____
   _____

# Depression

*"There are wounds that never show on the body that are deeper
and more hurtful than anything that bleeds."*

~ Laurell K. Hamilton

Veterans will consider deployment, disappointments, and biological and other factors in depression. They will talk about accepting help as a sign of strength, not a stigma. The participants will discuss challenges of digging out of the pits of despair and ways to draw upon internal strengths to develop resilience. Participants will engage in personal reflection and discuss ways to identify suicide risks and suicide prevention techniques.

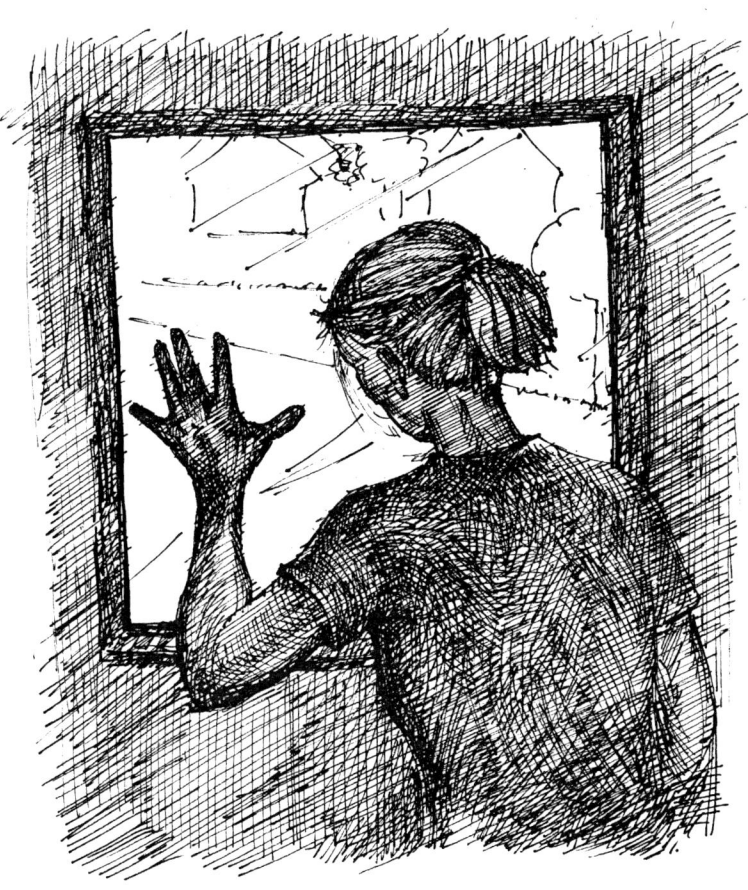

# High Hopes and Dark Days
# Facilitator's Guide

## Measureable Behavioral Objectives

**Veterans will ...**
- Identify the positive aspects of military experience.
- Determine possible disappointments related to their military experience.
- Check possible symptoms they are experiencing, noting situational and biological factors.
- Identify warning signs and actions to prevent suicide.
- Discuss their attitude toward getting help, (stigma or a sign of strength).
- Make an appointment and document time, date and address, (if mental health treatment is warranted).

## Introduction

1. Before the session begins, read this guide and the reproducible pages.
2. Decide on one of the interactive variations or the traditional approach (below).
3. Photocopy reproducible pages for participants but retain them until after the introduction.
4. Ask participants to brainstorm reasons they enlisted; a volunteer lists reasons on board.
5. Ask, *"If there are so many positives, why are many veterans depressed?"* List ideas on board.
6. Explain that they will be addressing ways to cope with depression.

## Activity

1. Distribute the reproducible pages.
2. Take turns reading the Education and Assessment portion aloud.
3. Encourage group members to check applicable boxes as they are read.
4. Discuss the importance of professional intervention if they are depressed or suicidal.
5. Allow time to complete the written Insight and Empowerment questions.
6. Encourage participants to share their responses.

## Conclusion

- Participants share what helped in the past when they were sad, and how those methods might help them now.

## Interactive Variation-Teams

1. Divide veterans into teams, one or a few topics per team (do not yet distribute the reproducible pages). Topics: Positives of Military Service, Negatives of Military Service, Signs of Depression and Suicidal Ideation, Causes of Depression, Stigma versus Strength Regarding Getting Help, Sources of Help for Emotional Problems and Substance Abuse.
2. Each team has paper and elects a leader to list their team ideas as they brainstorm regarding their topic.
3. After about ten minutes the group reconvenes; leaders share their teams' ideas with the whole group.
4. Distribute the reproducible pages and discuss any points the teams may have missed.
5. Encourage participants to complete the written portions at this time or for homework.

EDUCATION AND ASSESSMENT

# High Hopes and Dark Days

**Individuals have lofty reasons and high hopes for joining the military service: patriotism, serving their country, making a difference, carrying out family traditions, leaving the world better than they found it.**

Economic incentives exist: higher salaries than many civilian jobs, increments, bonuses; career opportunities; health insurance; housing; and educational assistance for service people and families.

With all of the above advantages, there are drawbacks: leaving loved ones and the comforts of home; harsh environments and strict rules; facing life and death daily; and returning home to possible financial problems and poor labor market. After the honeymoon period post-deployment, life's realities set in. Returning to life as you knew it is not probable: veterans and family members have changed; family dynamics are different; the job outlook is possibly bleak.

**Veterans may fall into a depressive state. Many symptoms are listed below. Check those that apply to you:**

- ❑ Sad, empty or irritable mood most of the time; no sense of peace.
- ❑ Diminished interest or pleasure in activities you formerly enjoyed including hobbies and sex.
- ❑ Decreased or increased appetite and weight loss or gain.
- ❑ Sleeping too much or too little compared to your normal pre-service sleep patterns.
- ❑ Either restlessness or extreme inactivity, observable by others.
- ❑ Fatigue for no real reason; lack of energy.
- ❑ Feelings of worthlessness or intense guilt, hopelessness and/or despair almost daily.
- ❑ Poor concentration, indecisiveness, feeling like you cannot think clearly.
- ❑ Recurrent thoughts of death, contemplation of suicide.
- ❑ Trouble functioning in social, occupational or other areas because of your symptoms.
- ❑ Medical exam ruled out physical illnesses or impairments.
- ❑ Digestive or other physical problems that your doctor states have no medical cause.
- ❑ Thinking nothing matters; being pessimistic.
- ❑ Difficulty loving self or others, loss of faith, decline in personal ethics.

- Be aware that grief and loss may elicit similar symptoms but depression lasts longer than the usual cycle of grief (which is individualized).
- Be aware that substance abuse may cause depression, or may be the result of depression.
- Example: the highs of cocaine or methamphetamine are followed by crashes; the rosy glow of drunkenness is followed by an irritable, restless hangover; some people self-medicate, using substances for a *feel good quick fix* instead of appropriate treatment.
- Additionally, some people have double trouble: two free-standing disorders - depression and addiction.
- Grief and loss, substance abuse and dual diagnoses are covered in other chapters.
- Spiritual support for grief and loss and treatment for sobriety is imperative, in conjunction with therapy and medication for depression.

*(Continued on the next page)*

EDUCATION AND ASSESSMENT

# High Hopes and Dark Days (continued)

**Causes of depression include situations such as:**

- Combat and other life-altering events; the aftermath of daily dangers.
- Separation, divorce, relational problems; unresolved grief and loss.
- Financial problems, unemployment, inadequate education or skills not appreciated by employers.
- Dealing with your partner's resentment due to increased responsibilities in your absence.
- Returning a different person, to a changed family, and adapting to new roles.

**Genetic and biological propensities.** A medical exam is needed to explore physical factors. Sometimes there is no apparent cause, but possibilities such as the following warrant evaluation:

- Chemical imbalances in the brain.
- A family history of depression.
- Nutritional and hormonal reasons.

**Other emotional conditions in addition to depression:**
A physician in conjunction with a licensed therapist will provide diagnosis and therapy. Medications will be prescribed if needed. You can help yourself by using cognitive changes, problem solving skills and coping skills.

Numerous resources exist for veterans and families for crisis intervention and treatment, and help with related issues including finances, legal aid, education, employment, substance abuse, work stress, divorce, grief and loss, housing and health assistance, etc.

## Suicidal Ideation

**If you are thinking about suicide, with a plan and a means to carry it out, call 911 or your local Emergency Services number, the National Suicide Prevention Lifeline/Veteran's Crisis Line, 1-800-273-8255 (TALK), or go to your nearest hospital Emergency Room.**

- Depression and substance abuse contribute to suicidal ideation.
- Being under the influence of meds or illegal substances can lead to reckless driving or overdosing.
- Professionals will take you seriously without condemnation or belittling if you acknowledge suicidal ideation.

INSIGHT AND EMPOWERMENT

# High Hopes and Dark Days

**Please answer the questions below.**

1. How were your high hopes upheld by the military experience?

2. In what ways have you been disappointed by your service or its aftermath?

3. What situational conditions contribute to your likelihood of experiencing depression?

4. What internal or biological factors are potential sources of depression for you?

5. From among the symptoms that apply to you from the checklist, which are most troublesome?

6. If grief and loss are issues, what are you doing to address those (spiritual counsel, support groups)?

7. If you suffer from substance abuse, what are you doing to seek recovery?

8. If you are suicidal with a plan and a way to act on it, what will you do to seek crisis intervention?

9. What will you do to seek help for any vague suicidal thoughts?

10. For some, a stigma exists regarding mental illness. Others seek help as a sign of strength. What is your attitude toward emotional challenges and getting help?

11. If you do not need immediate 911 assistance, please write the phone number you will call for Behavioral Health evaluation and treatment, (from your insurance card, or from your primary care MD referral, or from your Veteran's Administration or County Mental Health program):

12. Please dial the number now, make an appointment, record the time, date, and the address; if you are already in treatment, please write your next appointment information:

VETERANS: SURVIVING AND THRIVING AFTER TRAUMA

# Foxholes and Hope
# Facilitator's Guide

## Measurable Behavioral Objectives
**Veterans will ...**
- Link foxholes, black holes, other figurative *holes* with depression.
- State ways to stop the downward spiral and emerge from the *pits*.
- Determine false benefits they seem to get from their depression.
- Determine ways their trials have strengthened them.
- Identify actions they will take to improve their moods and outcomes.
- Apply quotes related to depression and hope to their lives and plan recovery-related measures.

## Introduction
1. Before the session, preview this guide and the reproducible pages.
2. Decide on one of the interactive variations or the traditional approach (below).
3. Photocopy reproducible pages but retain them until after the introduction.
4. You or a volunteer draw a picture of a foxhole on the board.
5. Ask participants to guess what the drawing represents.
6. Ask them to brainstorm thoughts about foxholes and holes in general.
7. Ask them to compare foxholes and holes to depression.
8. Explain they will be applying words of wisdom about holes, depression and hope to their lives.

## Activity
1. Distribute the reproducible pages.
2. Take turns reading the Education portion aloud.
3. Allow time to complete the written Insight and Empowerment questions.
4. Encourage participants to share their responses.

## Conclusion
- Ask participants to share the most helpful concept they learned at the session.

## Interactive Variations
- Ask participants to take turns reading the Insight and Empowerment questions and answering aloud.
- Ask participants to pair up with peers, read the questions to each other, record their partner's responses, then share with the group if they wish.

## Participants at the Board
1. After reading the Education portion aloud, tell participants to turn over their pages and put down pencils or pens.
2. Using a Master Copy, they take turns going up to the board, each person putting a quote (or two or three depending on instructions on the reproducible pages) on the board.
3. The person at the board reads the quote aloud, then asks the questions to peers and leads a discussion.
4. After all quotes have been discussed, people may then write their own reactions on their pages, (probably for homework if group time is limited).

EDUCATION & INSIGHT AND EMPOWERMENT

# Foxholes and Hope

## Education
- **Foxhole:** a small pit dug during action to provide individual shelter against hostile fire. Its purpose is protection at that moment. Some remain in a pit of depression long after combat, isolated, withdrawn, hiding from danger, cramped, falsely safe.
- **Black hole:** a region in time and space whose gravitational field is so strong that nothing which enters it, not even light, can escape. When depressed, you can feel sucked down by a vacuum, like you will never see the light of day.

## Insight and Empowerment
**Ponder the words of wisdom about holes and hope and apply them to your recovery:**

*It is good to follow the first rule of holes – if you are in one, stop digging.*
~ Dennis Healy

1. What are the signs that you are in a hole?

2. What have you been doing to dig in deeper?

3. How have you stopped digging?

4. What are you doing to climb out?

5. How will you prevent getting into a black hole?

*The gem cannot be polished without friction, nor can man be perfected without trials.*
~ Chinese Proverb

1. What have been your friction events and trials?

2. How have they polished you?

INSIGHT AND EMPOWERMENET

# The Tide Will Turn

**Consider the next three quotations to make sure you want to get out of the hole:**

*I'll never forget how the depression and loneliness felt good and bad at the same time. Still does.*
~ Henry Rollins

*In a strange way I had fallen in love with my depression . . . I loved it because I thought it was all that I had. I thought depression was the part of my character that made me worthwhile. I thought so little of myself, felt I had such scant offerings to give the world, that the one thing that justified my existence at all was my agony.*
~ Elizabeth Wurtzel

*Suffering isn't ennobling; recovery is.*
~ Christiaan Barnard

1. Give an example of how your depression and/or loneliness felt both good and bad at the same time.
   _____
   _____

2. Elizabeth Wurzel, (quoted above), thought that her depression was all she had, that it justified her existence and made her worthwhile. What falsely positive things has your depression done for you?
   _____
   _____

3. In what healthy and productive ways can you obtain the benefits you seemed to get from your depression?
   _____
   _____

4. How and why is it nobler for you to recover than to suffer?
   _____
   _____

*When you get into a tight place and everything goes against you, till it seems as though you could not hang on a minute longer, never give up then, for that is just the place and the time the tide will turn.*
~ Harriet Beecher Stowe

1. Share a time when you felt at your wits end when the tide turned in your favor:
   _____
   _____

2. What positive steps are you now taking to help yourself and to possibly stack the cards in your favor?
   _____
   _____

INSIGHT AND EMPOWERMENET
# What Lies Within?

***What lies behind us and what lies before us are tiny matters compared to what lies within us.***
~ Ralph Waldo Emerson

1. According to Emerson, what power is stronger than the past or future?
   _____
   _____

2. What inner strengths do you have or will you develop to overcome the past and fortify you for the future?
   _____
   _____


***If a dream should fall and break into a thousand pieces, never be afraid to pick up one of those pieces and begin again.***
~ Flavia Weedn

1. Share a dream that did not work out, one that is still important to you:
   _____
   _____

2. Describe the piece you can pick up:
   _____
   _____

3. What steps will you take to begin again?
   _____
   _____


***We must accept finite disappointment, but we must never lose infinite hope.***
~ Martin Luther King

1. Share a disappointment you must accept:
   _____
   _____

2. What steps are you taking to get and keep your hope?
   _____
   _____

# Reconnaissance and Resilience Facilitator's Guide

## Measurable Behavioral Objectives
**Veterans will ...**
- Define resilience and recognize its qualities within themselves.
- Acknowledge related attributes they have or are developing.
- Motivate themselves, naming things they enjoy and that give them a sense of accomplishment.
- Describe how to help others and give meaning and purpose to their own lives.
- Exemplify perseverance, prioritizing, organizing, flexibility, self-reliance and self-determination.
- Describe how they themselves are living proof that negative experiences need not cause irreparable damage.
- Relate the adversity in the poem Invictus to their lives; state how they are captains of their souls.

## Introduction
1. Before the session begins, read this guide and the reproducible pages
2. Decide on one of the interactive variations or the traditional approach (below).
3. Photocopy reproducible pages but retain them until after the introduction.
4. Write *Reconnaissance* on the board and elicit the definition.
5. Encourage participants to make analogies: they are on a reconnaissance mission against the enemy: depression; they will also investigate their own arsenal for the hidden weapon: resilience.
6. Write the word *Resilience* on the board and elicit the definition.
7. Encourage participants to share examples of their resilience.
8. Explain they will be further developing their resilience.

## Activity
1. Distribute the reproducible pages.
2. Take turns reading the Education and Assessment portion aloud.
3. Encourage group members to check the applicable boxes as they are read.
4. Allow time to complete the written Insight and Empowerment questions.
5. Encourage group members to share their responses to questions 1-8.

## Conclusion
- Read the poem Invictus (number 9) once aloud and then ask for one or two volunteers to read it to the group.
- Ask participants to share their responses to numbers 10, 11 and 12.

## Interactive Variations
- Ask participants to take turns reading the Insight and Empowerment questions aloud and answering orally.
- Ask participants to pair up with peers, read the questions to each other, record their partner's responses, then share with the group if they wish.

EDUCATION AND ASSESSMENT

# Reconnaissance and Resilience

**Reconnaissance is the process of obtaining information about a military position, activities, resources, etc., of an enemy or potential enemy. Resilience is the ability to spring back from and successfully adapt to adversity.**

- Your reconnaissance mission involves investigating the enemy: depression; you have learned of its pain, causes, and treatments, and are working on thought changing, problem solving, relationships, and, if relevant, chemical balance and sobriety.
- You have a powerful enemy you need to investigate, your ammunition for the investigation is your resilience.
- Keeping in mind that you have surmounted obstacles from basic training to grueling combat, draw upon your innate self-righting tendency; give yourself muscle.

**Consider the following quotes:**

*You say you are depressed – all I see is resilience. You are allowed to feel messed up inside and out. It doesn't mean you're defective – it just means you're human.*
~ David Mitchell

*I am a work in progress.*
~ Violet Yates

## Resilience involves the following attributes.
**Check the boxes that apply to attributes you have or are developing:**

- ❏ Expecting good outcomes regardless of risks
- ❏ Strengthening under stress, optimism regarding your buoyancy or ability to bounce back
- ❏ Building a support system
- ❏ Believing you can handle feelings and cope
- ❏ Making realistic plans and working toward goals
- ❏ Undertaking self-discovery and self-control after a crisis
- ❏ Building self confidence after honestly appraising personal strengths and weaknesses
- ❏ Willing to seek help and to self-disclose
- ❏ Seeing yourself as a survivor versus victim
- ❏ Sharing your strength, knowledge and hope to help others
- ❏ Knowing unfortunate experiences need not become unbearable problems
- ❏ Recognizing and accepting what cannot be changed
- ❏ Acting in adversity versus becoming immobilized, unless watching and waiting are warranted
- ❏ Visualizing an improved mood and a better life
- ❏ Taking care of your body, mind, emotions, spirit and soul
- ❏ Feeling gratitude, being glad to be alive despite death and destruction around you
- ❏ Finding meaning in your life: how can you use your experience to better your community and society?

INSIGHT AND EMPOWERMENT

# Reconnaissance and Resilience

**Answer the following questions to rev-up your Resiliency Factor**

1. When depressed, you lack desire to do things you used to enjoy. Think about what you liked to do for fun, or because it gave you a sense of accomplishment. If you wait until you feel like doing these, you may wait forever. Often, motivation comes after the action. List at least two enjoyable activities and two accomplishment-oriented activities you need to engage in:
   _____
   _____

2. Finding meaning and purpose for your life began when you joined the military. Some remain in the Reserves or National Guard, continuing to serve part-time; some return to civilian life exclusively and feel lost at first. How can your accomplishments in the military, and/or things you can do to help people, give meaning to your life?
   _____
   _____

3. It is important to set goals and plan steps toward them. You need perseverance, priorities, organization, and flexibility. Some rigid people want to *jump ship* at the first sign of turbulence. Share examples of these situations from your recent past, present or immediate future:
   a. Stick to a goal and plan despite set-backs.
   _____

   b. Honor priorities or revise them as needed.
   _____

   c. Organize a *Things To Do list* and cross off accomplishments.
   _____

   d. Change methods to reach your goal when new information is revealed or when situations swerve beyond your control.
   _____

4. Seeing the glass half-full versus half-empty is imperative; loss, change, pain, etc., are part of your military experience. In a crisis you can create a catastrophe, or use it as an opportunity for insight and growth; turn lemons into lemonade. List at least three positives regarding your current challenges:
   _____
   _____

5. Self-reliance is crucial; having supportive friends and family and finding a support system of veterans and families and other external helpers makes bouncing back easier. Because people are fallible and not always available, self reliance is required. Share a time your self-reliance carried you through a tough time.
   _____
   _____

6. How can you tap into your self-sufficiency to move you through current hurdles?
   _____

7. Self-Determination allows you to use your free will, to do what you believe in despite destructive criticism from others. Give a recent or current example of adhering to your principles.
   _____
   _____

8. How can you prove that negative experiences need not cause irreparable damage?
   _____
   _____

*(Continued on the next page)*

## INSIGHT AND EMPOWERMENT

# Reconnaissance and Resilience *(Continued)*

9. Ponder the following poem:

### Invictus

Also known as …I.M.R.T. Hamilton Bruce (1846-1899)
By William Ernest Henely (1849-1903)
Composed circa 1875

*Out of the night that covers me,*
*Black as the Pit from pole to pole,*
*I thank whatever gods may be*
*For my unconquerable soul.*

*In the fell clutch of circumstance*
*I have not winced nor cried aloud.*
*Under the bludgeonings of chance*
*My head is bloody, but unbowed.*

*Beyond this place of wrath and tears*
*Looms but the Horror of the shade,*
*And yet the menace of the years*
*Finds, and shall find, me unafraid.*

*It matters not how strait the gate,*
*How charged with punishments the scroll,*
*I am the master of my fate:*
*I am the captain of my soul.*

10. Describe ways the poet speaks to you including how your experiences are similar and how you are the captain of your soul.
    _____
    _____
    _____
    _____
    _____
    _____

11. What other special words or phrases did you encounter?
    _____
    _____
    _____
    _____

12. How do these words or phrases apply to your present situations?
    _____
    _____
    _____
    _____

VETERANS: SURVIVING AND THRIVING AFTER TRAUMA

# Sabotage Suicide Facilitator's Guide

## Measurable Behavioral Objectives

**Veterans will ...**
- Rate themselves on military and general risk factors for suicide.
- Verbalize the importance of telling someone about their suicidal thoughts and state sources of immediate assistance.
- Read statements regarding suicide prevention, including examples of defeated and survivor thoughts for each.
- State defeated thoughts and replace them with survivor ideas.
- State feelings and actions evolving from the defeated and survivor thoughts.
- Develop a twenty-four hour plan to stay alive.
- Analyze and apply life-promoting quotations to their lives.

## Introduction

1. Before the session begins, read this guide and the reproducible pages.
2. Decide on one of the interactive variations or the traditional approach (below).
3. Photocopy the reproducible pages but retain them until after the introduction.
4. Ask if anyone has ever felt suicidal, or known anyone who was suicidal.
5. Encourage participants to brainstorm reasons why service people might feel suicidal.
6. You or a volunteer list reasons on the board.
7. Explain that the most important action for a suicidal person to take is seek help.

## Activity

1. Distribute reproducible pages.
2. Take turns reading the Education and Assessment pages aloud.
3. Encourage participants to check applicable boxes as they are read.
4. Allow time to complete the written Insight and Empowerment questions.
5. Encourage participants to share their answers through number 14.

## Conclusion

- Encourage them to share their responses to the quotations (numbers 15 and 16).

## Interactive Variations

- Ask participants to take turns reading the Insight and Empowerment questions aloud and answering orally.
- Ask participants to pair up with peers, read the questions to each other, record their partner's responses, and share with the group if they wish.

EDUCATION AND ASSESSMENT

# Sabotage Suicide

**Suicide has emerged as a serious problem among veterans, and National Guard and Reserve members, even if they were never in combat.**

The military is redoubling efforts to prevent these deaths, but the stigma of asking for help stops many service members from life-saving treatment.

**Check the risks that apply to you:**

- ❑ Embarrassment in seeking mental health help.
- ❑ Relationship or romantic problems such as a Dear John letter or divorce.
- ❑ Money problems.
- ❑ Family problems.
- ❑ Substance abuse.
- ❑ Return from first deployment.
- ❑ Fear of disciplinary action, if remaining in the service.
- ❑ Fear of losing a rank or being discharged.
- ❑ Believing it is all over.
- ❑ Remorse about messing up.
- ❑ Viewing problems as unsolvable.
- ❑ Gender identity.
- ❑ Sexual orientation.
- ❑ Different culture.
- ❑ Long shifts and hard conditions.
- ❑ Depression, PTS(D), emotional or physical problems.
- ❑ Social isolation.
- ❑ Access to lethal weapons.


- The list could go on and on. Women as well as men, older people as well as youth, college students as well as service members, are also at risk.
- Men are at particular risk because women are more likely to seek help by expressing their emotions.
- If you are male, recognize it is macho to save your life, for your own sake, for your family, for your country, for all who will benefit from your strength in the future.
- If you are female, empower yourself to choose life.
- If your military experience contributed to your feeling suicidal, it is not your fault. You were caught in horrendous situations that most people never face in a lifetime.
- You need to be aware of signs within yourself and peers.
- Service members have been saved because buddies saw the signs and disabled their weapons.
- You might save another veteran, or by disclosing your suicidal ideation, be saved.

*(Continued on the nest page)*

EDUCATION AND ASSESSMENT

# Sabotage Suicide (Continued)

**Check the factors that apply to you:**
- ❑ Hopelessness; impulsive or aggressive tendencies.
- ❑ History of physical or sexual abuse, especially in childhood.
- ❑ History of family suicides, or your own prior attempts.
- ❑ Thinking about and talking about suicide.
- ❑ Planning, such as giving away possessions, making a will.
- ❑ Obtaining poison, a gun, a supply of medications for overdose, etc.
- ❑ Recent humiliation, failure of a relationship or loss of prestige.
- ❑ Reluctance to get help.
- ❑ Thinking you can't stop the pain, would be better off dead, have no way out, etc.
- ❑ Problems overeating or not eating enough.
- ❑ Problems sleeping too much, sleeping restlessly, not sleeping enough.
- ❑ Problems at work.
- ❑ Loss of enjoyment of any activities.
- ❑ Having financial issues.
- ❑ Feeling purposeless, worthless, trapped, desperate; believing life is not worth living.
- ❑ Extreme guilt, feeling like a burden to others.
- ❑ Thinking no one understands or cares.
- ❑ Inability to live in your own skin; to deal with your pain; feeling you are at the end of your rope.
- ❑ Hearing voices telling you to harm or kill yourself.

**If you are thinking about suicide, with a plan and a means to carry it out, call 911 or your local Emergency Services number, the National Suicide Prevention Lifeline/Veteran's Crisis Line, 1-800-273-8255 (TALK), or go to your nearest hospital Emergency Room.**

DEPRESSION

INSIGHT AND EMPOWERMENT
# Sabotage Suicide

Negative defeated thoughts could cause your death.
Replace them with positive but realistic survivor concepts.
See the statements below and the accompanying defeated and survivor examples.
Share your own defeated and survivor thoughts.

1. **The stigma of mental illness stops many people from seeking life-saving assistance.**
   Defeated: *People will think I'm crazy or weak if I need help.*
   Survivor: *My self-preservation instinct tells me to reach out to a lifeline.*
   Defeated: _____
   Survivor: _____

2. **Secrets kill.**
   Defeated: *It's nobody's business that I'm suicidal.*
   Survivor: *I'll tell a trusted person, seek out a professional, or call 911 or a Hotline.*
   Defeated: _____
   Survivor: _____

3. **Suicidal thoughts are usually helpless and hopeless.**
   Defeated: *I see no way out.*
   Survivor: *I can learn to solve my problems or accept situations and move forward.*
   Defeated: _____
   Survivor: _____

4. *Suicide is a permanent solution to a temporary problem.* ~ Phil Donahue
   Defeated: *Life is not worth living like this.*
   Survivor: *I'll give my thoughts, feelings and situation time to change.*
   Defeated: _____
   Survivor: _____

5. **Current catastrophes are smaller and more manageable than they appear.**
   Defeated: *This is the worst that could happen; I cannot recoup.*
   Survivor: *I'll picture myself surviving and thriving five years from now.*
   Defeated: _____
   Survivor: _____

6. **Reasons for living keep people alive through tough times.**
   Defeated: *No one cares; there is no reason to face this pain.*
   Survivor: *My family, friends, buddies, or Higher Power care; or… I choose to care about my life, to make my life count for something or somebody I don't yet know.*
   Defeated: _____
   Survivor: _____

*(Continued on the next page)*

INSIGHT AND EMPOWERMENT

# Sabotage Suicide *(Continued)*

7. **People honor contracts.**
   Defeated: *I can't promise anybody anything.*
   Survivor: *I promise myself, my Higher Power, or loved ones that I will watch and wait.*
   Defeated: _____
   Survivor: _____

8. **Drugs, alcohol, and over-using prescribed medications increase suicide risk.**
   Defeated: *I'll drink myself into oblivion; then I won't feel the pain.*
   Survivor: *I need to be sober and think straight in this crisis.*
   Defeated: _____
   Survivor: _____

9. **Safe environments save lives.**
   Defeated: *I have guns, knives, a vehicle, and pills in case I decide to act on suicidal thoughts.*
   Survivor: *I'll hand over my weapons, car keys, etc. to someone until I trust myself.*
   Defeated: _____
   Survivor: _____

10. **Distractions, activities, being with people, and helping others prolong life.**
    Defeated: *I am obsessed with suicide; nothing brings me joy; I can't be with people.*
    Survivor: *I can do things I used to enjoy, go to a safe place, and try to help others.*
    Defeated: _____
    Survivor: _____

11. **A twenty-four hour plan helps people live one day at a time.**
    Defeated: *I don't know or care what I do from one minute to the next.*
    Survivor: *I'll make a twenty-four hour safety plan and stick to it.*
    Defeated: _____
    Survivor: _____

12. **People can be forgiven and can heal from grief and loss.**
    Defeated: *I deserve to die for what I did; or…I can't live without my partner, etc.*
    Survivor: *With help, I can attempt amends, forgive myself, accept the loss, etc.*
    Defeated: _____
    Survivor: _____

13. **Look back at your defeated thoughts and list at least three feelings and three actions that could result from that negativity:**
    _____
    _____
    _____

14. **Look back at your survivor thoughts and list at least three feelings and three actions that could result from that positivity:**
    _____
    _____
    _____

*(Continued on the next page)*

## INSIGHT AND EMPOWERMENT

# Sabotage Suicide *(Continued)*

15. Consider this quotation:
    ***Anyone desperate enough for suicide ... should be desperate enough to go to creative extremes to solve problems: elope at midnight, stow away on the boat to New Zealand and start over, do what they always wanted to do but were afraid to try.*** ~ Richard Bach

    a. Brainstorm outrageous creative solutions to your problems:

    b. What (positive activity) have you always wanted to do but were afraid to try?

16. Consider this quotation:
    ***The most authentic thing about us is our capacity to create, to overcome, to endure, to transform, to love and be greater than our suffering.*** ~ Ben Okri

    a. What is something positive that you can create?

    b. What will you overcome?

    c. What will you endure?

    d. What will you transform?

    e. How will you transform yourself?

    f. What will you love?

    g. Who will you love?

    h. How will you be better than your suffering?

# Guilt

*"Guilt should be a momentary pang to spur one into corrective action. Anything longer is wasted, and worse, selfish."*

~ Mark Belletini

Sources of combat-related guilt and ways to substitute productive for unproductive guilt will be addressed. Facilitator will encourage participants to make amends and correct wrongs when possible and to work toward spirituality and self-forgiveness. Veterans will discuss ways to change regret into reform.

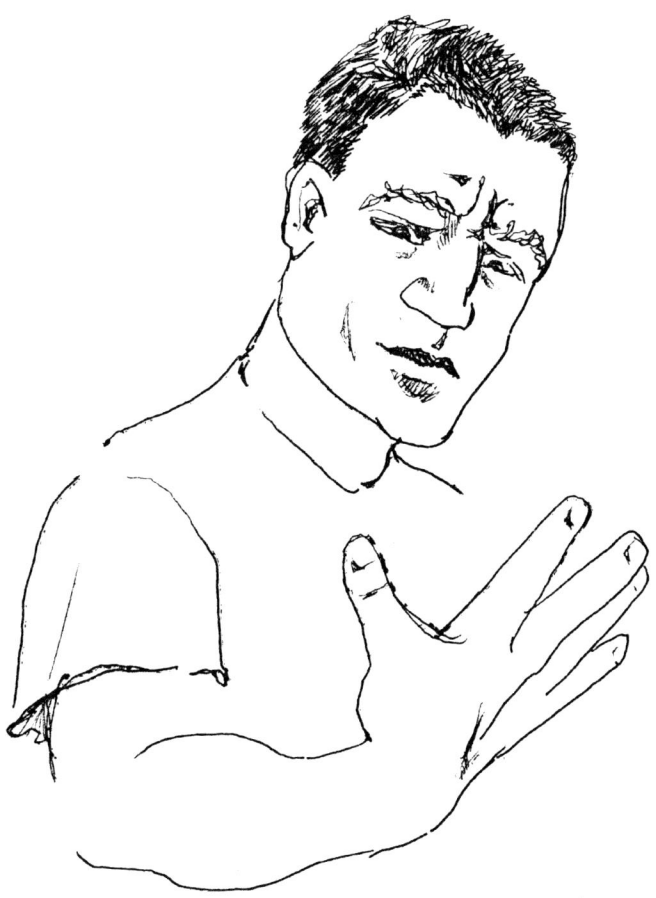

VETERANS: SURVIVING AND THRIVING AFTER TRAUMA

# Is All Fair in War? Facilitator's Guide

## Measurable Behavioral Goals
**Veterans will ...**
- Identify common sources of combat-related guilt.
- Identify specific situations and actions causing their guilt.
- Describe aspects of the event beyond their control.
- State what they would say to comfort a buddy suffering the same remorse.
- Share what they wished they had done differently.
- Determine to whom to acknowledge their wrongdoing.
- Determine from whom to receive forgiveness.
- Write a letter of forgiveness to themselves.
- Identify the self-destructive behaviors they have inflicted on themselves, possibly due to believing they deserve punishment and pain.
- Determine ways they can make amends and do good deeds now and in the future.

## Introduction
1. Before the session begins, read this guide and the reproducible pages.
2. Decide on one of the interactive variations or the traditional approach (below).
3. Photocopy reproducible pages but retain them until after the introduction.
4. Write on the board the two quotations: *All is fair in love and war*, and *The rules of fair play do not apply in love and war*.
5. Encourage a discussion in response to this question: *Do you believe these statements are true? Why or Why not?*
6. Explain that whether or not they agree with the quotations, many veterans are guilt-ridden, which worsens depression and has led to self-destructive acts including suicide.

## Activity
1. Distribute the reproducible pages.
2. Take turns reading the Education and Assessment portion aloud.
3. Encourage participants to check applicable boxes as they are read.
4. Allow time to complete the written Insight and Empowerment questions.
5. Encourage participants to share their responses.

## Conclusion
- Explain that a conscience or inner critic is often developed in childhood. Ask them to share the benefits and drawbacks of their inner critic.
- Benefits may involve keeping us from wrongdoing and righting our wrongs; drawbacks exist if we expect perfection or beat-up on ourselves versus developing compassion and self-forgiveness.

## Interactive Variations
- Ask participants to take turns reading the Insight and Empowerment questions aloud and answering orally.
- Ask participants to pair up with peers, read the questions to each other, record their partner's responses, then share with the group if they wish.

EDUCATION AND ASSESSMENT & INSIGHT AND EMPOWERMENT

# Is All Fair in War?

## Education and Assessment

***All's fair in love and war,*** per Francis Edward Smedley, and ***The rules of fair play do not apply in love and war,*** per John Lyly, are controversial statements.

They suggest following your heart in love regardless of consequences and behaving very viciously to gain victory in war and love. They imply that extreme matters require extreme measures; that we are exonerated for actions at the height of emotion; that judgment and insight are impossible during such times.

However ...

- Veterans brought up to never kill feel guilt about killing the enemy or civilians.
- Friendly fire deaths elicit even more remorse.
- Buddies being murdered and maimed while others are saved cause survivor guilt.
- Many veterans inflate their own power, blaming themselves for situations beyond their control.
- Some feel they deserve to be punished and suffer because of an action or inaction.
- Combat-related guilt has led to many suicides.

Studies done with Viet Nam combat veterans apply today. They cited reasons for guilt.
Check the boxes that apply to your sense of guilt:

- ❑ Taking human lives, performing violent acts.
- ❑ Losing prior moral values, thereby permitting you to commit atrocities.
- ❑ Killer – Self identity, getting high on the power of life and death.
- ❑ Guilt about past and present violent acts and wishes, causing self-destructive symptoms and more guilt; believing your suffering is proper punishment for combat deeds.
- ❑ Inability to control persistent violent urges or behaviors; possibly leading to suicide attempts and homicidal fantasies.
- ❑ Believing you are evil, that you sold out to the devil.
- ❑ Turning against or away from your prior spirituality and faith, being plagued with demoralization and doubt; being spiritually and morally numb.
- ❑ Believing you have been part of a morally corrupt system.

## Insight and Empowerment

1. Summarize the situation and your actions that are causing your feelings of guilt:
   _____
   _____

2. What aspects of the event were not within your control, (such as following orders)?
   _____
   _____

3. With the information and resources you had at that time, how did you do the best you could?
   _____
   _____

4. What was your intention at the time of the decision or action?
   _____
   _____

## INSIGHT AND EMPOWERMENT

# Is All Fair in Love and War? *(Continued)*

5. With hindsight, what do you wish you had done differently?

6. What would you tell your best buddy if he or she suffered guilt from this situation?

7. Explain how your standards are too high for the reality of the situation, or why your standards are appropriate for you.

8. If your standards are unrealistically high, write a statement making them match the real world:

9. If you truly believe you fell short, with whom can you share your remorse?

10. From whom can you receive forgiveness? (Possibly other veterans who have *been there and done that*, or a spiritual or religious leader or your Higher Power.)

11. Elaborate on the following:
    a. How high is your Higher Power?

    b. Is your Higher Power more judging and punitive or more merciful and forgiving?

    c. If your Higher Power forgives you, what is keeping you from forgiving yourself?

12. If you believe you have lost your old faith, what might a new-found, more mature spirituality and faith look like for you based on the hard-won wisdom of your war experience?

13. Write a letter to yourself, forgiving yourself, and stating how you will avoid self-destruction.

14. Consider the following words of wisdom:

    ***Chronic remorse, as all the moralists agree, is not a most undesirable sentiment. If you behaved badly, repent, and make what amends you can and address yourself to behaving better the next time. On no account brood over your wrongdoing. Rolling in the muck is not the best way of getting clean.***
    ~ Aldous Huxley

    Have you been *rolling in the muck*?

    How can you make amends?

15. Consider this quote:

    ***Every man is guilty of all the good he did not do.*** ~ Voltaire

    What positive actions can you take now and in the future, what *good* will you do?

# Painful or Productive Guilt?
# Facilitator's Guide

## Measurable Behavioral Objectives
**Veterans will …**
- Refute painful, non-productive thoughts about their guilt.
- Replace those thoughts with realistic and productive thoughts.
- Identify lessons learned from mistakes.
- Describe attributes and actions that improve their self-concepts.
- State how to prevent making the same errors in the future.
- Describe ways to turn their regret into reform.

## Introduction
1. Before the session begins, read this guide and the reproducible pages.
2. Decide on one of the interactive variations or the traditional approach (below).
3. Photocopy the reproducible pages but retain them until after the introduction.
4. Write on the board, *I'll never forgive myself.*
5. Ask participants, *"What's wrong with that statement?"* Elicit that it is a misery-making thought that does nothing to help them or to right a wrong.
6. Write on the board, *Painful or Productive Guilt?*
   Encourage a discussion of the differences between guilt that hurts and guilt that helps.

## Activity
1. Distribute the reproducible pages.
2. Take turns reading the Education portion aloud.
3. Allow time to complete the written Insight and Empowerment questions.
4. Encourage participants to share their responses through number 11.

## Conclusion
- Ask participants to either recite their responses to number 12, or if time permits, ask them to write on the board and receive peer feedback.

## Interactive Variations
- Ask participants to take turns reading the Insight and Empowerment questions aloud and answering orally.
- Ask participants to pair up peers, read the questions to each other, record their partner's responses, then share with the group if they wish.

## Brainstorming
- Ask participants to brainstorm pain-producing guilt-ridden thoughts while you or a volunteer write them on the board.
- Ask participants to refute each idea and make it productive while you or a volunteer write the revisions under each of the negative thoughts on the board.

EDUCATION & INSIGHT AND EMPOWERMENT

# Painful or Productive Guilt?

## Education and Assessment

- Painful guilt cuts to your core, causing self-loathing and destructive behavior: drugs and alcohol, self injury, suicidal
- ideation, lashing out at others, nightmares, lack of sleep, etc.
- Productive guilt motivates you to better yourself and the world.
- Changing your thoughts results in healthier feelings and healing actions.
- Consider the examples below and make the suggested changes.

## Insight and Empowerment

See the italicized erroneous examples and then, answer the questions regarding your regretful behavior and situation:

1. *It's all my fault* is a fallacy because other factors and folks were involved.
   What circumstances and people played a role?
   _____
   _____
   _____

2. *I always do wrong* is invalid because you do many right things.
   Share the wrong behavior you did once or sometimes:
   _____
   _____
   _____

3. Share at least two of your actions that you do well, that make you proud or give you peace:
   _____
   _____
   _____

4. *My life is a mess because of my mistakes* is untrue; you probably have learned a lot.
   Share at least two lessons learned from your mistakes:
   _____
   _____
   _____

5. *I hate myself* may seem true now, but you probably don't, and if you do, you can learn to love yourself. Admittedly, you did some things you dislike. List at least two attributes that increase your-self-worth. Consider that you were created for a purpose, that you have abilities and aspirations.
   _____
   _____
   _____

6. *Everyone thinks I'm a loser* is untrue because all people do not think the same and you do not know what others think. You are projecting onto others what you think about yourself. List at least two of your winner qualities.
   _____
   _____
   _____

*(Continued)*

INSIGHT AND EMPOWERMENT)

# Painful or Productive Guilt? *(Continued)*

7. *If only I hadn't done that … I should have, could have …* are useless thoughts. You cannot turn back the clock. Describe what you are doing now so you won't repeat the same errors:

   _____
   _____
   _____

8. *I'll never change* is untrue; you are evolving daily. You must accept what cannot be changed about yourself in the past; you can change yourself now. What three changes are you now making to improve yourself, to enlighten other veterans, to help your family, to rectify wrongs?

   _____
   _____
   _____

9. Consider the wisdom of this quote:

   > ***When one door closes, another opens; we often look so long and so regretfully upon the closed door that we do not see the ones which open for us.***
   >
   > ~ Alexander Graham Bell

   Describe the door that is open for you now and how to make the most of the opportunity:

   _____
   _____
   _____

10. Consider the wisdom of this quote:

    > ***Remorse begets reform.***
    >
    > ~ William Cooper

    What reforms are you making?

    _____
    _____
    _____

11. Consider the wisdom of this quote:

    > ***It's not what you are, it's what you don't become that hurts.***
    >
    > ~ Oscar Levant

    What are you becoming?

    _____
    _____
    _____

12. Compose your own words of wisdom regarding moving forward from guilt and regret:

    _____
    _____
    _____
    _____

# Grief

*"The pleasure of remembering had been taken from me, because there was no longer anyone to remember with. It felt like losing your co-rememberer meant losing the memory itself, as if the things we'd done were less real and important than they had been hours before."*

~ John Green

**V**ETERANS WILL ANALYZE AND APPLY the wisdom of *In Flanders Fields* (John McCrae) to their lost comrades, and determine how they, as survivors, might carry the torch. They will identify their own responses to the stages of grief and loss to ease their transition to the healing level.

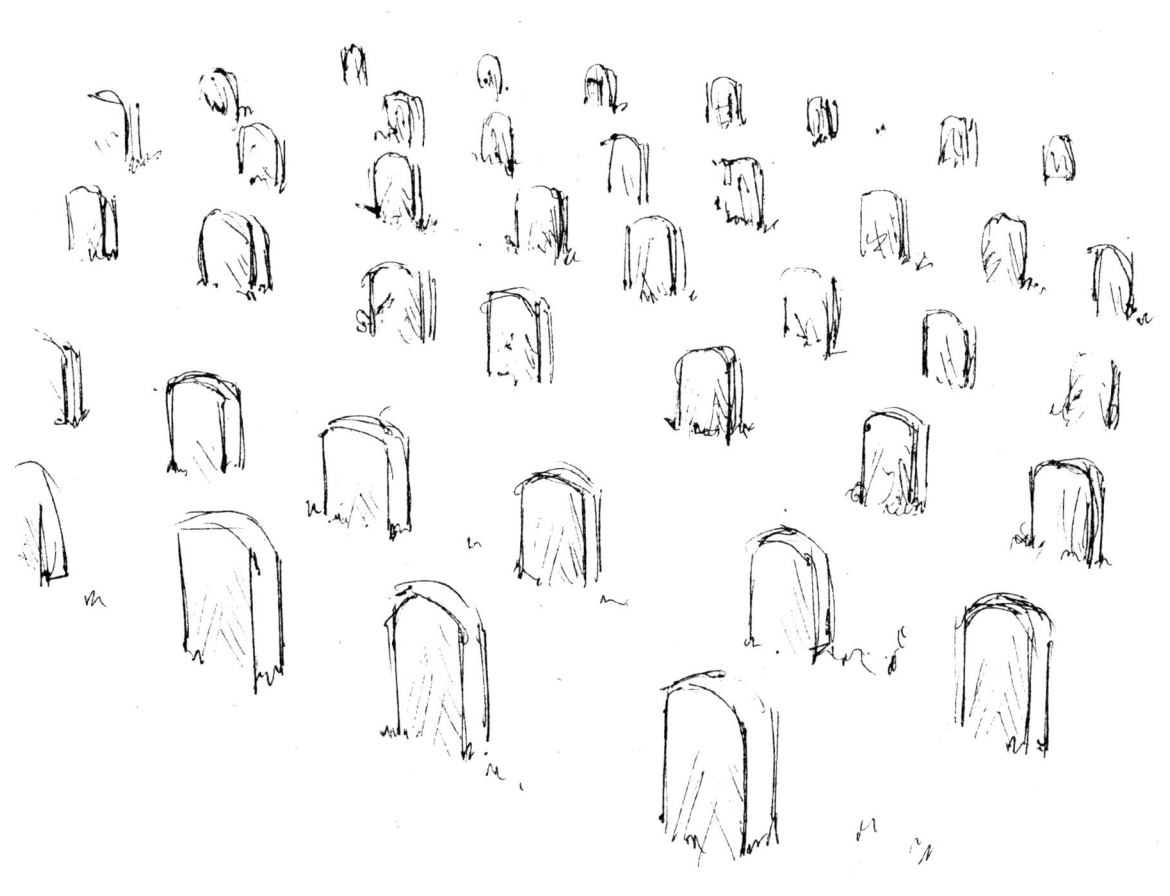

# Shock and Awe
# Facilitator's Guide

## Measurable Behavioral Objectives

**Veterans will ...**
- Apply their experiences to possible stages, acknowledging that grief is an individualized process.
- Identify warning signs that warrant professional referrals.
- Read symptoms and coping skills of survivor guilt.
- Describe ways to help themselves reach reconstruction and acceptance.
- State name, address, date, and phone number for their Veteran's Administration or other appointments, if needed.

## Introduction

1. Before the session begins, read this guide and the reproducible pages.
2. Decide on one of the interactive variations or the traditional approach (below).
3. Photocopy the reproducible pages but retain them until after the introduction.
4. Write on the board *Shock and Awe*.
5. Ask group members what it means in military terms and the generic meaning of the words.
6. Ask about shock and awe as first reactions to death of a combat buddy or loved one. Elicit that survivors often feel overwhelmed, and may lose their will to go on.

## Activity

1. Distribute the reproducible pages.
2. Take turns reading the Education and Assessment portion aloud.
3. Encourage participants to check the Warning Signs as they are read.
4. Allow time to complete the written Insight and Empowerment questions.
5. Encourage participants to share their responses.

## Conclusion

- Emphasize the importance of seeking treatment from their Veteran's Administration, mental health professional or spiritual advisor if they have warning signs or prolonged pain.

## Interactive Variations

- Ask participants to take turns reading the Insight and Empowerment questions aloud and answering orally.
- Ask participants to pair up with peers, read the questions to each other, record their partner's responses, then share with the group if they wish.

EDUCATION AND ASSESSMENT

# Shock and Awe

**Shock and Awe is a military doctrine of rapid dominance; the use of overwhelming power and spectacular force to paralyze the enemy's perception of the battlefield and destroy their will to fight.**

- Shock, disbelief and denial are usually the first reactions to death.
- Awe involves fear and dread, natural reactions to loss, especially sudden death.
- You may grieve the loss of your former identity, innocence after combat, a dream if you change careers due to emotional or financial problems, etc.
- The grief process is individualized. Stages have been theorized, but people do not go through all the same stages and no specific time frames exist.

**Elizabeth Kubler-Ross named five stages of grief:**

1. Denial, a defense mechanism, that buffers immediate shock.
2. Anger, we resent the pain and loss, then are guilty about being angry.
3. Bargaining, *If only I had been better toward them*; or if they are still alive, we tell our Higher Power, *If they are saved I promise ...*
4. Depression, sadness, about practical concerns and the loss.
5. Acceptance, new normal, easier after a long illness or advanced age; harder to accept when a soldier dies in the prime of life.

***GriefWork ~ Healing from Loss* lists three markers along the Healing Pathway:**

1. Shock - The reality of the loss has not sunk in.
2. Disorganization - The reality of the loss is real.
3. Reorganization - Rebuilding a satisfying life - a New Normal.

EDUCATION AND ASSESSMENT

# Shock and Awe

## Survival Guilt compounds grief among many veterans
- Some ask, *why wasn't it me who got hurt or killed.*
- Some take responsibility or blame, *it's my fault.*
- Some think, *the dead person deserved to live and I deserved to die.*

## Survival Guilt is helped if you act accordingly:
- Admit your feelings.
- Realize survival guilt is common, but not comfortable.
- Seek others who understand, veterans, support groups, family.
- Mourn the loss, possibly by a ceremony or some other way to commemorate the person's life.
- Act and live as they would have advised; make a contribution, hold a fundraiser, give blood, time, and energy to the causes they believed in.

## Warning Signals
Some symptoms are dangerous and require professional help.
**Place a check mark next to the symptoms of depression or complicated grief that apply to you.**
- ❏ Thoughts of harming or killing yourself or others.
- ❏ Inability to trust yourself or others.
- ❏ Persistent belief that you deserve(d) to die.
- ❏ Inability to function months after the death; cannot perform at work or school; unable to care for children or household responsibilities.
- ❏ Severe depression and hopelessness about the future; feeling worthless.
- ❏ Inability to eat or sleep or take care of personal health and hygiene.
- ❏ Feelings of extreme guilt, rage or bitterness.
- ❏ Substance abuse, including taking higher than recommended doses of prescribed medications.
- ❏ Extreme physical reactions like nausea, aches and pains, lowered immunity.
- ❏ Very slow thinking, speech and body movements.
- ❏ Seeing or hearing things that are not there.
- ❏ False beliefs that the person still lives; searching for them, or thinking you recognize them in familiar places.
- ❏ Envy toward others who are not suffering, or not caring about others.

**Answer the Insight and Empowerment questions on page 101 that apply to you.
Anticipating an upward turn, restoration, or acceptance may hasten your progress.**

GRIEF

INSIGHT AND EMPOWERMENT

# Shock and Awe

1. Share your initial shock and denial.

2. Share your anger regarding the injury or death.

3. Share your guilt and your survivor guilt if applicable.

4. With whom did you bargain, and how?

5. Share your depression and sadness about practical aspects of your loss such as changes in financial and other responsibilities.

6. Reflect upon loneliness.

7. How did you or do you plan to bid your buddies farewell?

8. How do you plan to memorialize and celebrate their life?

9. Tell about your upward turn or how you will know you are reaching it.

10. How did you or do you plan to reconstruct yourself and your life?

11. Share thoughts about your acceptance.

12. What are your hopes for yourself and your life for the future?

13. Who are people in your support system and how can you expand your support system?

14. What spiritual practices comfort you?

15. Write a letter to your lost buddy and say things you never said before.

16. A journal, scrapbook, photo album, or memory box may help. Share your experiences or plans regarding these techniques.

17. Draw, write a song, poem, or paragraph about your loss and recovery.

18. Making a collage or sculpture may also help. State your ideas:

19. Laughter lifts your mood. Describe a funny situation you shared.

20. If you have the any of the warning signals or if these interventions do not help, you may need medication, or grief counseling from a spiritual advisor or therapist. Write name, address, date, and phone number regarding your Veteran's Administration or other doctor:

# Carry the Torch Facilitator's Guide

## Measurable Behavioral Objectives
**Veterans will …**
- Express emotions evoked by poem, *In Flanders Fields* by Dr. John McCrae.
- Describe memories about the deceased, and what the deceased might say to them.
- Make individualized analogies regarding larks, the foe and their torch.
- Share how they will not break faith with the deceased.

## Introduction
1. Before the session begins, read this guide and the reproducible pages.
2. Decide on one of the interactive variations or the traditional approach (below).
3. Photocopy the reproducible pages but retain them until after the introduction.
4. Ask if anyone has heard or read the poem, *In Flanders Fields*.
5. Ask about their recollections of the poem.
6. Explain that the Dead are supposedly speaking; it is their voices we hear.

## Activity
1. Distribute the reproducible pages.
2. Read the poem aloud.
3. Ask for two volunteers to read it in unison.
4. Listeners can use highlighters to focus on words or phrases personally meaningful.
5. Ask for initial thoughts, feelings and interpretations.
6. Discuss the information above the poem, about the author, life and death.
7. Allow time to complete the written Insight and Empowerment questions.
8. Encourage participants to share their responses.

## Conclusion
- Encourage participants to find more war poems and share them during the next session.
- Encourage participants to write poetry regarding related topics; remind them it need not rhyme.

## Interactive Variations
- Ask participants to take turns reading the Insight and Empowerment questions aloud and answering orally.
- Ask participants to pair up with peers, read the questions to each other, record their partner's responses, then share with the group if they wish.

## Teams
1. Group members break into two teams.
2. Each elects a recorder to write their team members' responses.
3. Teams discuss the questions and the recorder writes all answers.
4. Teams brainstorm regarding the analogies, larks, foe and torch.
5. Both teams re-convene and the recorders share their responses.
6. Teams give feedback to each other.

EDUCATION & INSIGHT AND EMPOWERMENT

# Carry the Torch

## Education

Dr. John McCrae, a lieutenant colonel and physician in the Canadian army, wrote this poem in 1915, after witnessing a friend die. He writes from the perspective of the dead, in their voice. The crosses row on row, suggest large numbers of graves. Today, as then, throngs who lived, loved and were loved, now lie.

### In Flanders Fields by Dr. John McCrae

*In Flanders fields the poppies blow*
*Between the crosses, row on row,*
*That mark our place; and in the sky*
*The larks, still bravely singing, fly*
*Scarce heard amid the guns below.*
*We are the Dead. Short days ago*
*We lived, felt dawn, saw sunset glow,*
*Loved and were loved, and now we lie,*
*In Flanders fields.*
*Take up our quarrel with the foe:*
*To you from failing hands we throw*
*The torch; be yours to hold it high.*
*If ye break faith with us who die*
*We shall not sleep, though poppies grow*
*In Flanders fields.*

## Insight and Empowerment

This poem and other pieces of literature are open to the reader's interpretation. No right or wrong explanations exist. Respond to the questions based on your understanding and how the images of this poem apply to you.

1. Depending on the feelings and visions this evoked, please draw, write, meditate, pray…

2. Poppies, red in color, ironically grew in blood-soaked fields. Today they represent remembrance. How do you remember the person or people you lost?

3. The larks have been considered symbols of beauty and freedom contrasted with the guns and graves below. Some see larks, still bravely singing, as people with perseverance and courage. What do the larks mean to you?

4. The Dead speak in this poem. What would your deceased person say to you?

5. Taking up the quarrel with the foe has many interpretations: continue the war? fight the enemy? The foe may be war itself, or intangibles like prejudice, hate, ignorance, etc. What foe will you fight?

6. The torch may be an object of pride. Describe about whom or of what your person was the most proud.

7. What does the torch in this poem represent?

8. Handing over a torch symbolized transferring a duty. What will you do to carry on the person's responsibilities, beliefs and aspirations?

9. How will you not break faith with the person?

# Substance Abuse

*"Do not let your fire go out, spark by irreplaceable spark, in the
hopeless swamps of the approximate, the not-quite, the not-yet, the not-at-all.
Do not let the hero in your soul perish, in lonely frustration for the life you deserved,
but have never been able to reach. Check your road and the nature of your battle.
The world you desired can be won. It exists, it is real, it is possible, it is yours.*

~ Ayn Rand

Veterans will focus on possible tendencies to abuse substances, and determine their biological and environmental risks, including combat and post-deployment stresses. They will consider ways to decrease denial and to identify defense mechanisms. They will make analogies between the substance and a forbidden romance and change from glamorizing alcohol or drugs to focusing on the rewards of recovery. Veterans facing dual diagnoses (emotional and addictive conditions) will practice ways to implement physiological, psychological and cognitive coping techniques.

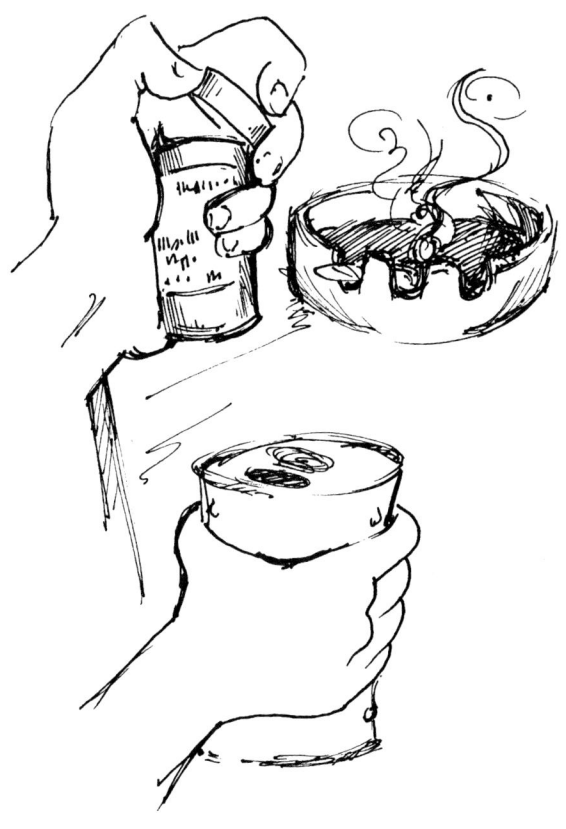

# Nature and Nurture
# Facilitator's Guide

## Measurable Behavioral Objectives
**Veterans will ...**
- Identify possible symptoms of substance abuse and dependence from possible indicators.
- State their risks from biological and environmental factors.
- Answer questions to decrease denial and increase insight.
- Rate themselves regarding barriers to receiving help.
- State whether and how they have used tactics to delay getting help.
- Share their pros and cons regarding treatment types and support groups.
- Read options for accessing treatment and support groups.
- Answer questions to encourage inspiration and insight from a quotation.

## Introduction
1. Before the session begins, read this guide and the reproducible pages.
2. Decide on one of the interactive variations or the traditional approach (below).
3. Photocopy the reproducible pages but retain them until after the introduction.
4. Write on the board, *Heredity versus Environment, Nature versus Nurture.*
5. Ask group members to brainstorm inherited traits as you list them on the board.
6. Ask group members to list environmental factors that influence who we are as you list them on the board.
7. Explain that professionals have discussed and debated whether nature or nurture causes or contributes most to substance abuse and addiction.
8. Encourage group members to discuss and debate their thoughts and opinions.
9. Explain that current beliefs are that both nature AND nurture impact individuals.

## Activity
1. Distribute the reproducible pages.
2. Take turns reading the Education and Assessment portion aloud.
3. Encourage participants to check applicable symptoms as they are read.
4. Allow time to complete the written Insight and Empowerment questions.
5. Encourage participants to share their responses through number 7.

## Conclusion
- Ask participants to read the quotation aloud, then share their responses to the questions.

## Interactive Variations
- Ask participants to take turns reading the Insight and Empowerment questions aloud and answering orally.
- Ask participants to pair up with peers, read the questions to each other, record their partner's responses, then share with the group if they wish.

EDUCATION AND ASSESSMENT

# Nature and Nurture

**Veterans are at risk for substance abuse and dependence related to the strain of multiple deployments, combat exposure and other factors. Reckless driving, domestic strife and emotional problems often accompany substance abuse.**

- No one likes to give up what has given them pleasure.
- Alcohol and drugs are double-edged swords; one side seemingly subdues your problems, the other worsens them.
- Substances at first elicit euphoria; eventually you need those substances to feel *normal*.
- Substance abuse and addiction are chronic, progressive and potentially fatal.

**Check the following items that apply to you:**

- ❏ Failure to fulfill your roles and responsibilities at home, work, school.
- ❏ Use in situations in which it is hazardous; driving or operating machinery under the influence.
- ❏ Legal problems such as DUI, arrests for disorderly conduct.
- ❏ Continued substance use despite interpersonal and other problems; arguments about the substance with partner and family; fights when under the influence.
- ❏ Need for increased amounts to achieve the desired effect and diminished effects with the same amount.
- ❏ Suffering the opposite effect of the substance when it wears off: hyperactivity, nausea, anxiety after a calming agent; *crashing*, prolonged sleep after a stimulant.
- ❏ Taking the same or a similar substance for relief such as a drink the morning after.
- ❏ Use of larger amounts or over a longer period than was intended.
- ❏ Persistent desire or unsuccessful attempts to cut down or control your use.
- ❏ Spending a lot of time in obtaining, using and recovering from the substance.
- ❏ Giving up important occupational, social or family activities because of substance use.
- ❏ Continued use despite problems caused or worsened by the substance.

The above checked boxes are indicators that you may be abusing or dependent upon substances.

EDUCATION AND ASSESSMENT

# Nature and Nurture

Why can some people use a substance socially, take it or leave it, while others go *hog wild* for it? Nature versus Nurture arguments attempted to explain addiction. The current trend is Nature **and** Nurture.

Check the boxes that apply to you:

Nature-Biology: your genes may pre-dispose you to addiction.
- ❑ Parents, grandparents, other blood relatives have abuse or addiction issues.
- ❑ Family members or you have suffered from emotional problems.

Nurture-Development: early life and adolescence may have laid groundwork.
- ❑ You saw substances abused by caregivers and role models.
- ❑ You gave in to peer pressure in your teens, drank or used with your friends.
- ❑ You were abused emotionally, physically or sexually.

Nurture-Environmental Stress adds *fuel to the fire*.
- ❑ You were exposed to combat or other stressful conditions.
- ❑ You have a diagnosis of PTSD or TBI.
- ❑ You have been subject to multiple deployments.
- ❑ You have other stresses regarding finances, family, employment, etc.

The CAGE Assessment for Alcohol Abuse is the quickest easiest questionnaire, and applies to other substances as well as alcohol.

**Check the boxes if your answer is YES:**
- ❑ **C** = Have you felt the need to **C**ut down on your drinking?
- ❑ **A** = Do you feel **A**nnoyed by people complaining about your drinking?
- ❑ **G** = Do you ever feel **G**uilty about your drinking?
- ❑ **E** = Do you ever drink an **E**ye-opener in the morning to relieve the shakes?

Additional clues follow.

**Check the boxes if your answer is YES:**
- ❑ Do you lie to people about your substance use?
- ❑ Have you tried switching from one drink or drug to another?
- ❑ Do you need the substance just to feel *normal* or to function?
- ❑ Do you dislike places where your substance of choice is unavailable
- ❑ Do you drink or use beforehand?
- ❑ Do you create opportunities to meet friends at a bar or throw parties?
- ❑ Do you panic when your supply is low or carry it around with you?
- ❑ Do you have blackouts and no memory of your actions after intoxication?
- ❑ Do you do things under the influence that you later regret?
- ❑ Have you been advised to make an appointment with a physician or counselor?
- ❑ Do you deliberately visit different physicians and pharmacies to get more prescriptions?

## INSIGHT AND EMPOWERMENT

# Nature and Nurture *(Continued)*

**Barriers to getting help are listed below. Check boxes that apply to you:**
- ❑ Unaware of the need for treatment.
- ❑ Unaware of local options.
- ❑ Long waits for Veteran's Administration or other initial appointments.
- ❑ Unsure what costs are covered by insurance, or options for the uninsured.
- ❑ Long distances to V.A. or other treatment center.
- ❑ Stigma – fearing negative labels in records as mentally ill or an addict.
- ❑ Family unwilling or unable to be involved in treatment.
- ❑ Fear of the unknown, thinking you will give up freedom.
- ❑ Other reasons _____

Defense mechanisms and other tactics prevent and delay recovery. Examples are italicized.
Share your use of these defense mechanisms:

1. **Denial**: You lie to yourself: *I don't have a problem. I can quit any time.*
   _____

2. **Rationalization**, making it acceptable: *The doctor prescribed my pain pills, so they must be ok. I need extra energy from speed for work.*
   _____

3. **Blaming** is common: *My family doesn't understand. If my spouse didn't start arguments, I'd be ok.*
   _____

4. **Procrastination**: *I can't deal with it now. I'm going through too much. I'll do it after I finish school, or get discharged, or…*
   _____

5. **Reluctance**: *Do I really want to give up what's been my best friend, my escape from reality, my comforter, entertainer, energizer?*
   _____

6. **Excuses** are found: *I can't go into treatment because I have to work, go to school, and take care of the kids.* (How well are you working, studying, or taking care of kids when intoxicated and withdrawing?)
   _____

7. **Indecision**: *Will I keep doing the same thing and expecting different results? This no longer works for me, what now?*
   _____

As you start your journey toward insight and healing, consider these words:

**Believe more deeply. Hold your face up to the light, even though for the moment you do not see.**

~ Bill Wilson

Describe what you believe more deeply:
_____
_____

How are you holding your face up to the light?
_____
_____

# Romancing or Recovering? Facilitator's Guide

## Measurable Behavioral Objectives
**Veterans will …**
- Rate themselves regarding indications of a romance with a substance.
- Read about the importance of thought changing, and potential rewards of recovery.
- State how they will stop mentally flirting with the substance.
- Describe consequences of their drinking or drugging.
- Identify compelling rewards for being clean and sober.
- Share indicators of their probable powerlessness over the substance.
- State ways their lives have become unmanageable.
- Identify ways a rehabilitation program might help them.
- Share what they can become in sobriety; how placing sobriety first helps.
- Identify their ammunition for this battle.

## Introduction
1. Before the session begins, read this guide and the reproducible pages.
2. Decide on one of the interactive variations or the traditional approach (below).
3. Photocopy the reproducible pages but retain them until after the introduction.
4. Ask a volunteer to walk in the room with sunglasses.
5. Ask, *"How will these affect his or her vision?"*
6. Write on the board, *Rose colored glasses*, and ask the meaning of the term. Elicit that they color or distort our vision making things look better.
7. Write on the board *Romancing* and ask what it means to be romancing a person or idea. Elicit: excitement, anticipation, remembering the good times and minimizing the bad, etc.
8. Ask if it is possible to love something rather than someone; elicit the power of pleasure from alcohol and drugs.
9. Explain they will be re-thinking their true love.

## Activity
1. Distribute the reproducible pages.
2. Take turns reading the Education and Assessment portion aloud.
3. Encourage participants to check applicable items as they are read.
4. Allow time to complete the written Insight and Empowerment questions.
5. Encourage participants to share their responses through number 11.

## Conclusion
- Ask participants to take turns reading at least one of the quotations aloud and sharing their answer to the questions, (numbers 12, 13, and 14).

## Interactive Variations
- Ask participants to take turns reading the Insight and Empowerment questions aloud and answering orally.
- Ask participants to pair up with peers, read the questions to each other, record their partner's responses, then share with the group if they wish.

EDUCATION AND ASSESSMENT

# Romancing or Recovering?

**Do you have a romance with a substance? Check the boxes that apply to you:**
- ❑ Do you eagerly anticipate spending time with it?
- ❑ Does it make you feel good?
- ❑ Do you have fond memories of it?
- ❑ Are you obsessed with it?
- ❑ Do you live for the next time you can be with it?
- ❑ Have you continued your relationship despite destruction?
- ❑ Do you meet in secret?
- ❑ Does it mean more to you than other loves in your life?
- ❑ Would you lay down your life for it?

Anything that makes you feel so good is hard to give up. Think of the consequences instead of only the rosy glow. The more you flirt with the thought of drinking or drugging, the more likely you are to follow through.

**Do not think that what your thoughts dwell on does not matter. Your thoughts are making you.**

~ Bishop Steere

Human nature validates that positive rewards are more powerful than negative consequences. If punishments worked, people would stop boozing after their first hangover, there would never be a second DUI charge (*driving under the influence*), and stimulant users would stop using after their first *coming down* episode.

Finding and focusing on rewards of recovery are paramount. Instead of thinking about your loss (of the substance), think about your gains in terms of the following. Check the boxes related to rewards you seek:
- ❑ Mental and physical health.
- ❑ Recognizing versus hiding from reality.
- ❑ Improved relationships.
- ❑ Improved finances.
- ❑ Improved performance at home, work, or school.
- ❑ Improved spirituality or serenity.
- ❑ Improved intellect.

Do not expect a quick fix:

- Mentally, you may feel worse at first; anxieties after tranquilizing effects wear off or depression after a high will eventually pass.
- Physical discomforts from the shakes to nausea will subside; you will be healthier.
- Finances should show profits quickly; less spent on the substance.
- Depending on whether the substance *seemed* to help you function, your performance will eventually be better without the lethargy of crashing and the sickness of hangovers.
- Explore rehabilitation programs through referrals from your physician or mental health professional. You will learn the impact of the substance on your life, find strength to change, receive help from spirituality, a sponsor, (personal mentor or coach), and other recovering people.

INSIGHT AND EMPOWERMENT

# Romancing or Recovering?

1. Describe ways your substance has been like a lover:

2. Romancing and glamorizing the substance in your mind leads to inevitable cravings; how can you stop the daydreams as soon as they start?

3. Describe five consequences of your drinking or drugging. How were you and others affected?

4. Identify five compelling rewards that would be an incentive for you for be clean and sober:

5. What are three signs that suggest you are powerless or have difficulty giving up the substance?

6. List three ways the substance makes your life unmanageable:

7. Tell three ways a sponsor, other recovering people or support persons might help you:

8. Give examples of two problems remaining or worsening despite a substance-related escape:

9. Relationships may not improve immediately; describe two people close to you and how their roles will change when you are clean and sober:

10. Your substance was your lover and may have been a god; who or what will replace it and how?

11. Your thinking may seem fuzzy at first. What activities will you seek to improve your concentration and memory?

12. *The important thing is this: To be able at any moment to sacrifice what we are for what we could become.*
    ~ Charles du Bois

    When you sacrifice what you are in addiction, what can you become?

13. *The older I get, the more wisdom I find in the ancient rule of taking first things first — a process which often reduces the most complex human problems to manageable proportions.*
    ~ Dwight D. Eisenhower

    How can you place sobriety first and how will that help you manage your problems and your life?

14. *You might have to fight a battle more than once to win it.* ~ Margaret Thatcher

    If you have tried before to be clean and sober, or if this is your first attempt, describe your new ammunition:

SUBSTANCE ABUSE

# Dual Battles Facilitator's Guide

## Measurable Behavioral Objectives

**Veterans will ...**
- Rate themselves regarding mental health and substance-related factors.
- Share past results and current efforts regarding medications, therapy, peer support and self help for mental health and sobriety.
- Change self-defeating to wellness-promoting thoughts.
- State their activities to promote mental health and a clean and sober lifestyle regarding expression, assertion, inspiration, nutrition, exercise, recreation, intellectual development, stress management, sleep and relaxation, problem solving, support system and productive activity.

## Introduction

1. Before the session begins, read this guide and the reproducible pages.
2. Decide on one of the interactive activities or the traditional approach below.
3. Photocopy the reproducible pages but retain them until after the introduction.
4. Write *DUAL* on the board and ask its meaning. Elicit that it means double or twofold.
5. Write *DUEL* on the board and ask its meaning. Elicit that it means a battle.
6. Explain that many veterans face double trouble: emotional and substance abuse problems.
7. Encourage participants to brainstorm reasons as a volunteer lists them on the board.
8. Tell them they can learn how to fight both battles.

## Activity

1. Distribute the reproducible pages.
2. Take turns reading the Education and Assessment portion aloud.
3. Encourage participants to check applicable items as they are read.
4. Allow time to complete the written Insight and Empowerment questions.
5. Encourage participants to share their responses.

## Conclusion

- Ask participants to share whether they think their emotions led to substance abuse or their substances led to emotional problems. Or do they have two independent but interdependent problems?
- Acknowledging that twofold treatments are needed for dual issues, ask them to identify ways that improving each condition helps the other.

## Interactive Variations

- Ask participants to take turns reading the Insight and Assessment questions aloud and answering orally.
- Ask participants to pair up with peers, read the questions to each other, record their partner's responses, then share with the group if they wish.

© 2013 WHOLE PERSON ASSOCIATES, 101 WEST 2ND ST., SUITE 203, DULUTH MN 55802 • 800-247-6789

EDUCATION AND ASSESSMENT

# Dual Battles

Statistics from studies of Viet Nam, Iraq and Afghanistan veterans show that many have co-occurring disorders, often PTSD or depression and substance abuse or dependence. If you have emotional and alcohol or drug problems, your physician may determine you have a dual diagnosis.

Combat stress has led to emotional reactions and self-medication with substances. Some veterans had biological propensities toward emotional problems or addiction. Combat worsened their condition(s). Others had no indicators for either disorder.

**Check the boxes that apply to you:**
- ❑ I have a family history of emotional problems.
- ❑ I have no family history of addiction.
- ❑ I had highs and lows or anxiety symptoms before I used alcohol or drugs.
- ❑ Alcohol or drugs helped my symptoms at first.

If you checked all or most of the above boxes, your emotional issues might be resolved with medications, talk therapy and coping skills. Once your moods are stabilized, you might not turn to alcohol or drugs.

**Check the boxes that apply to you:**
- ❑ I have a family history of addiction.
- ❑ I have no family history of emotional problems.
- ❑ I had no highs or lows or anxiety symptoms before using alcohol or drugs.
- ❑ I had physical pain and was prescribed opiates and over-used them.
- ❑ I feel my worst when my substance wears off and, or use another substance to help withdrawal symptoms.

If you checked all or most of the above boxes, your substance use problems can be resolved with treatment. Once you are clean and sober for a period of time, your mood swings and anxiety might cease.

**Check the boxes that apply to you:**
- ❑ I have a family history of both emotional and addiction problems.
- ❑ It's hard to say whether emotional problems or substance abuse started first.
- ❑ I had several months clean and sober, but still had mood problems or anxiety.
- ❑ I was stabilized emotionally for months, but still craved alcohol or drugs.

If you checked all or most of the above boxes, you may have two free-standing conditions. You probably need medication, therapy and coping skills for the emotional symptoms, and chemical dependency treatment. In your case, one problem is not causing the other, but each compounds the other.

- The good news: if your physician says you have a dual diagnosis, you can find professional treatment, peer support and self-help from many sources.

SUBSTANCE ABUSE

INSIGHT AND EMPOWERMENT

# Dual Battles

See your physician. You may need medications, possibly to help your mood or sleep. Tell your doctor about substance abuse so addictive medications will not be prescribed. Never take another person's medications.

1. If you have a history of emotional issues and medications, what meds have and have not helped?
   _____
   _____

2. Fill in the boxes below:

| Name of Medicine | Purpose | Who Prescribed It? | Side Effects | Addictive Potential? |
|---|---|---|---|---|
| Ex: antidepressant | lift my mood | psychiatrist | drowsiness | no |
| | | | | |
| | | | | |
| | | | | |
| | | | | |
| | | | | |

3. If more than one physician is prescribing, they all need to know what you are taking, including over the counter medicines and herbal remedies, because of interactions. With whom do you need to share medication information?
   _____

4. Mixing alcohol or drugs with medicine is dangerous. If you did this, describe the results:
   _____

5. What are you doing now to make sure your medications work safely and optimally?
   _____

6. Medications may help addiction recovery. Share attempts at sobriety with medical monitoring, telling what has and has not helped:
   _____

7. Emotional issues are helped by therapy; you can process feelings about your military and other experiences; learn coping and problem solving skills. Share what has and has not helped you and why:
   _____

8. Recovery and rehabilitation programs help people remain clean and sober; share what has and has not helped you and why.
   _____

INSIGHT AND EMPOWERMENT

# Winning Dual Duels

1. Practice changing two self-defeating thoughts to wellness-promoting replacements. See example below.
   Negative: *I am a chronic relapser.* (This sets you up to fail.)
   Positive: *I am in recovery working on sanity and sobriety.* (This gives you hope.)
   Negative: _____
   Positive: _____
   Negative: _____
   Positive: _____

2. Coping skills, stress management, and lifestyle changes help mental health and sobriety. Share what you are doing or plan to do regarding the following:

   a. Expressing feelings through journaling, letters, or poetry, etc.:
   _____

   b. Expressing feelings through art, cartoons, collages, doodling, music, drama, etc.:
   _____

   c. Assertion, placing sanity and sobriety first; saying *No* as needed:
   _____

   d. Seeking serenity and inspiration from reading, meditation, nature, prayer, etc.:
   _____

   e. Proper nutrition for body and mind:
   _____

   f. Exercise/sports for body and emotions (raising levels of endorphins-feel good chemicals):
   _____

   g. Recreation, clean-sober fun:
   _____

   h. Mental gymnastics to keep intellect sharp, (puzzles, classes, etc.):
   _____

   i. Sleep-wake cycle stabilization:
   _____

   j. Relaxing through guided imagery, progressive muscle relaxation, deep breathing, etc.:
   _____

   k. Problem-solving skills, brainstorming, listing pros and cons, etc.:
   _____

   l. Support system, professionals and trustworthy family members and friends:
   _____

   m. Productive activity, school, work, volunteering, helping people or social causes:
   _____

3. Share whether your emotional problems led to self-medication with substances, or your substances led to emotional problems. Do you have two independent but interdependent problems?
   _____

4. Although twofold treatments are needed for dual issues, how does improving each condition help the other?
   _____

# Coping Skills

*"When we are no longer able to change a situation,
we are challenged to change ourselves."*

~ Viktor Frankl

V<small>ETERANS WILL IDENTIFY AND DISCUSS</small> ways to correct cognitive distortions, noting resultant changes in feelings and actions. They will apply techniques to challenge distorted thoughts and practice problem solving and solution-oriented skills. Self-expression is promoted via art, writing, music, movement, sports and reading to recreate themselves.

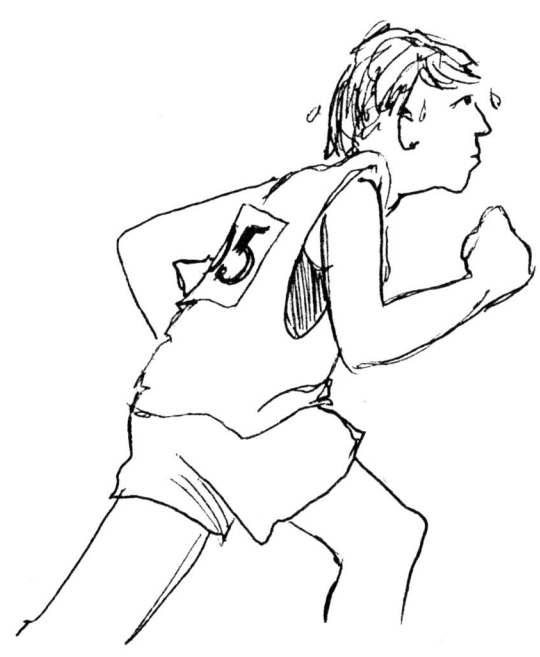

# Cognitive Counterforce Tactics Facilitator's Guide

## Measurable Behavioral Objectives

**Veterans will ...**
- Identify thought distortions; replace them with positive realistic thoughts.
- Note how feelings and actions change due to thought replacement.
- Use techniques to refute negative thought patterns.
- Change at least one unproductive behavior and note the accompanying change in feelings and thoughts.
- Practice shared responsibility to decrease guilt and shame.
- Apply relevant quotations to their thoughts and lives.

## Introduction

1. Before the session begins, read this guide and the reproducible pages.
2. Decide on one of the interactive variations or the traditional approach (below).
3. Photocopy the reproducible pages but retain them until after the introduction.
4. Ask if the group members have ever heard the expression to *fight fire with fire?*
5. Ask for their interpretations, and ask them to relate the expression to their thoughts. Elicit responses recognizing that we must fight distorted thoughts with corrected thoughts.
6. Write on the board and ask for interpretations: *Outlooks affect outcomes.*
7. Write on the board and ask for interpretations: *Fake it 'til you make it.*
Elicit that we can act our way into better thinking.

## Activity

1. Distribute the reproducible pages.
2. Take turns reading the Education and Assessment portion aloud.
3. Allow time to complete the written Insight and Empowerment questions.
4. Encourage participants to share aloud their responses through number 19.

## Conclusion

- Encourage participants to apply the quotations (number 20) to their lives and to share other words of wisdom they have heard or created themselves regarding this topic

## Interactive Variations

- Ask participants to take turns reading the Insight and Empowerment questions aloud and answering orally.
- Ask participants to pair up, read the questions to each other, record their partner's responses, then share with the group if they wish.

EDUCATION AND ASSESSMENT

# Cognitive Counterforce Tactics

Thought changing affects emotions and actions. Methods to change your thinking:

1. Identify and correct the thought distortions below.

| Thought Distortion | How to Change It | Negative Thought | Positive Thought |
|---|---|---|---|
| All or Nothing or Black and White | Substitute shades of gray or middle of the road. | Nothing good can come of it. | Surviving might strengthen me. |
| Overgeneralizing | Be more specific. | My wife cheated; you cannot trust women. | Some can be trusted and some cannot. |
| Mental Filter or Magnifying Negatives | Find some positives. | I saw death and the cruelty of human nature. | I saw some heroism. |
| Discounting or Minimizing positives | Focus on your attributes. | I did nothing right. | I did the best I could; I helped some people. |
| Jumping to Conclusions or Fortune Telling | Presume and predict favorable outcomes. | I will never get better. | I will improve with coping skills, and find faith. |
| Mind Reading | Decide your own opinion matters. | They are thinking the worst about me. | They may care about what I've been through. |
| Emotional Reasoning | Use your head not your feelings. | I'm depressed; my life isn't worth living. | I am going through tough times; I will find a purpose. |
| Shoulda-Coulda-Woulda; If only… | Know that the past cannot be changed. | I should have done it differently. | I learned from my mistakes. |
| Labeling | Stop stereotyping. | I'm a lost cause. | I am worth saving. |
| Blaming | Seek solutions. | It's all my (or their) fault. | How can we rectify the situation? |
| Catastrophizing | See a challenge. | This is impossible. | I will give it my best. |
| Excessive Self Criticism | Cut yourself some slack. | I can't bounce back. | It may take a while but I can emerge stronger. |
| Making Demands | Make requests. | Do it now! | Would you please consider doing this? |
| Self-Fulfilling Prophesy | Measure up to expectations. | I can't get out of debt. | I'll get financial advice and stick to a budget. |
| Personalizing | See the big picture. | It's my entire fault. | I had a part, but some situations were beyond my control. |

EDUCATION AND ASSESSMENT

# Cognitive Counterforce Tactics *(Continued)*

2. **Thought Replacement:** Substitute a more positive but realistic thought and note the change in feelings and actions. Example: Change *I'm at the end of my rope*, to *what I've been doing is not working. I'll try something different*. This conjures up hope and leads to action.

3. **Pros and Cons:** Negativity leads to misery; positive thinking leads to hope and problem-solving behavior.

4. **Examine the Evidence:** Weigh the facts. What is the statistical likelihood that everything will always go wrong, or that something is entirely your fault? Extenuating circumstances and fallible humans are involved.

5. **Reality Check:** Ask positive people if your ideas are realistic or distorted. Believe them!

6. **Experience and Experiment:** If you think, *I can't change*, think about past experience and ways you changed; experiment with changing something simple to prove you can.

7. **Best Buddy:** Talk to yourself as you would to a buddy. Be your own best friend, not your own worst enemy.

8. **Activity Replacement:** Act your way into better thinking and feeling. Help others. Rate your satisfaction in your efforts on a ten best scale. Compliment yourself for doing, regardless of your feelings.

9. **Per Cents:** Ask yourself the likelihood that something will turn out favorably. Instead of *I'll never get over it*, ask *what are the chances of some relief?* Any per cent is better than zero. See continuum example, showing a fifty percent likelihood of getting some relief.

```
   0%                      x=50% likelihood                    100%
Never get better                                         Recover for sure
```

10. **Watch Your Language:** Instead of negatives, use neutral terms. *I'm getting worse again*, causes panic; acknowledge, *some symptoms are recurring; I'll tell the doctor*. This is honest and action-oriented.

11. **Share Responsibility:** Instead of self-blame, *I killed people*, say *I followed orders to kill in a war zone; it was to kill or be killed*. You had few choices or independent decisions to make.

12. **Acknowledge and Accept:** Atrocities occurred; you fell short of your standards. Decide: *I gained strength and endured*. Resolve to use your experience to help yourself and others.

13. **Empower Yourself:** Ask yourself, *what can I do to improve the relationship?* Decide to listen carefully, communicate more openly, seek couples counseling, etc.

14. **Seek Spiritual Counsel:** Know you are valued, forgiven, have a purpose; can recover, hope, and love again. Find wisdom in literature, beauty in nature, joy in music, love in family, or whatever soothes your soul.

INSIGHT AND EMPOWERMENT

# Cognitive Counterforce Tactics

1. Complete the boxes below; see number 1 on Education and Assessment, page 119, for examples.

| Distortion | My Old Thought | My Corrected Thought |
|---|---|---|
| All or Nothing or Black and White | | |
| Overgeneralizing | | |
| Mental Filter | | |
| Minimizing the Positives | | |
| Jumping to Conclusions | | |
| Mind Reading | | |
| Emotional Reasoning | | |
| Shoulda-Coulda-Woulda: If only… | | |
| Labeling | | |
| Blaming | | |
| Catastrophizing | | |
| Self-Criticizing | | |
| Making Demands | | |
| Self-Fulfilling Prophecy | | |
| Personalizing | | |

## INSIGHT AND EMPOWERMENT

# Cognitive Counterforce Tactics: Negative → Positive

2. Fill in the boxes below to show how changing your thoughts from negative to positive will change your feelings and actions.

| Negative thoughts | Feelings resulting from the negative thoughts | Actions likely to result from the negative thoughts and feelings | Positive but realistic replacement thoughts | Feelings resulting from the positive thoughts | Actions likely to result from the positive thoughts and feelings |
|---|---|---|---|---|---|
| Example: The war ruined my life. | Hopeless and helpless. | Give up, drink, drug, attempt suicide. | I can make my life better. | Hopeful, empowered. | Ask for therapy; learn new coping skills. |
|  |  |  |  |  |  |

3. List the disadvantages of the negative thought in Negative → Positive.

4. List the advantages of the replacement thought in Negative → Positive.

5. Write a different negative thought that upsets you often.

6. Objectively examine the evidence for the truth of this statement. Explain if and how it is exaggerated or slanted and how it works against your peace and success.

7. Consider the thought you wrote in number 5, or another intrusive thought. Ask others you trust whether it is valid or distorted. Write their responses.

8. Write one of your troublesome thoughts below.

9. Refute the above thought based on your current growth, sharing why the thought is not true.

## INSIGHT AND EMPOWERMENT

# Cognitive Counterforce Tactics: Negative→Positive *(Continued)*

10. Describe a stress inducing situation that recurs frequently and elicits negative thinking.
    _____
    _____
    _____

11. Talk to yourself as you would to a best friend about the situation in number 10. Suggest positive ways to view the situation:
    _____
    _____
    _____

12. If you were not burdened by your military experiences, imagine what would you be doing and how you would be thinking and feeling at this point in your life.
    _____
    _____
    _____

13. Within the next day, act as if you were not burdened by your past. Do something you would have done before your trauma; act in a previously positive way; and then describe what you did, how you acted, and how you felt during and after the performance.
    What I did: _____
    How I acted: _____
    How I felt during the activity: _____
    How I felt immediately afterward: _____
    How do you feel now after *acting as if?* _____

14. In what upcoming challenge do you plan to *fake it 'til you make it?*
    _____
    _____
    _____

15. Think of an event that conjures up guilt or shame. Share the responsibility. Describe circumstances beyond your control and people involved who contributed to the incident.
    _____
    _____
    _____

16. Regarding your role in the event in number 15, what lessons have you learned and how have you changed in positive ways as a result of the unfortunate occurrence?
    _____
    _____
    _____

17. Think of an ongoing challenging situation in which your thoughts, feelings and actions need to change, a situation wherein you recently felt hopeless and helpless. Realistically appraise yourself and assign a per cent of possibility that you will improve:
    _____
    _____
    _____

## INSIGHT AND EMPOWERMENT

# Cognitive Counterforce Tactics: Negative→Positive *(Continued)*

18. What can you do to improve your thoughts, feelings and actions in this area of your life?

19. How can you enlist your faith or develop spiritual strengths to help you change and to improve the situation?

20. Apply at least three of the following quotations to your thinking patterns and your life:

*Change your thoughts and you change your world.* ~ Norman Vincent Peale

*We must become the change we want to see.* ~ Mahatma Gandhi

*Turbulence is life force. It is opportunity. Let's love turbulence and use it for change.*
~ Ramsay Clark

*There is nothing like returning to a place that remains unchanged to find the ways in which you yourself have altered.* ~ Nelson Mandela

*The universe is change; our life is what our thoughts make it.* ~Marcus Aurelius Antoninus

COPING SKILLS

# Problems Can Be Opportunities Facilitator's Guide

## Measurable Behavioral Objectives
**Veterans will …**
- Define their problem(s) that contribute(s) to emotional discomfort.
- Set specific, measurable goals and identify internal and external resources.
- Brainstorm solutions, weigh the pros and cons, select feasible options.
- List related steps, take action, and evaluate the effectiveness of their solution(s).
- Acknowledge improved attitudes and abilities as a result of their efforts.
- Determine what worked for them in the past and how to use those skills in current situations.
- Identify productive actions to meet their needs.
- Identify their constructive and destructive habits.
- State ways constructive habits will improve their relationships, moods and lives.

## Introduction
1. Before the session begins, read this guide and the reproducible pages.
2. Decide on one of the interactive variations or the traditional approach (below).
3. Photocopy reproducible pages but retain them until after the introduction.
4. Write on the board *Problems are only opportunities in work clothes* ~ Henri Kaiser.
5. Ask whether group members agree or disagree and discuss times their problems became opportunities.
6. Explain that group members will practice problem solving techniques.

## Activity
1. Distribute the reproducible pages.
2. Take turns reading the Education portion aloud.
3. Allow time to complete the written Insight and Empowerment questions.
4. Encourage participants to share their responses through number 19.

## Conclusion
- Encourage participants to share how they will use constructive habits (number 20).

## Interactive Variations
- Copy the Problem-Solution chart on the board (number 8).
- Ask participants to take turns sharing their problems while peers brainstorm solutions, pros and cons;
- A volunteer writes them in the chart's boxes on the board.
- Ask peers to help each other decide on Plans A and B (number 9).

EDUCATION & INSIGHT AND EMPOWERMENT

# Problems Can Be Opportunities

## Education

While chemical imbalances (treated with medication) and negative thinking (treated with thought changing) contribute to emotions, problems create havoc. Veterans face a slew of them, from employment issues, to finances, to housing, to relationships, etc.

*Problems are only opportunities in work clothes*, according to Henri Kaiser. Opportunities involve openings, breaks, prospects for a better you, an improved mood, a more effective way of life. Work involves effort and rewards.

Linking symptoms to situations, defining problems and goals, identifying and selecting options and evaluating your progress are basic aspects of Problem Solving.

An alternative is to focus on what's right in your life, what works for you, decisions about what has decreased problems in the past, and application of similar methods now.

Additionally, you can replace damaging attitudes and actions with caring and constructive habits and then reap relationship rewards, which will improve your mood.

## Insight and Empowerment

The following questions incorporate adaptations of the above therapies and/or philosophies.

1. What symptoms cause you emotional discomfort?

2. What situation or primary problem activates your distress?

3. When, where, and with whom does the problem usually occur?

4. What is a specific, measurable, and achievable goal for you regarding this issue?

5. What strengths do you have to help you? Describe specifics related to your experience, ability, motivation, creativity, etc.

6. What external resources can you tap into? Describe specifics including the people who can help, support groups, sources of information on the internet and elsewhere, professional assistance, etc.

*(Continued on the next page)*

INSIGHT AND EMPOWERMENT

# Problems Can Be Opportunities *(Continued)*

7. In your wildest imagination, conjure up possible solutions to a current problem. Use the back of this paper to complete your list, as you should need lots of time to dream and room to write!

   _____
   _____
   _____
   _____

8. Now cross off impossible solutions; list a few feasible ones in the table below, and fill in pros and cons.
   *Example:* Problem – *No one understands my trauma and suffering.*

| Solutions | Pros | Cons |
| --- | --- | --- |
| Ex: *Join the local veterans' club.* | *Other veterans know what I've been through; we share our problems.* | *I drink there and focus on my misery.* |
| Ex: *Join a different veterans' club.* | *They understand my pain and lobby Congress for better benefits.* | *It's ten miles farther to drive.* |

**Your Focus Problem**

| Solutions | Pros | Cons |
| --- | --- | --- |
|  |  |  |
|  |  |  |
|  |  |  |

9. Decide what you think is the best solution, Plan A or, in case Plan A doesn't work, Plan B.

   *Ex:* Problem – *No one understands my trauma and suffering.*
   Plan A – *Join a veterans' club that promotes programs to help survivors.*
   Plan B – *Get professional help for my emotions.*

   Your Focus Problem:

   _____
   _____

   Your Plan A

   _____
   _____

   Your Plan B

   _____
   _____

## INSIGHT AND EMPOWERMENT

# Problems Can Be Opportunities *(Continued)*

10. For your problem as noted in number 9, list the steps you need to take to complete Plan A.
    *Ex:* Plan A Steps for *Join a veterans' club*:
    ✓ Look online and in the phone book for local clubs.
    ✓ Try a few clubs; select the one that works toward improvements for service people and veterans.

    Your Plan A
    _____

    List the steps to complete Plan A
    ✓ _____
    ✓ _____
    ✓ _____
    ✓ _____

11. For your problem as noted in number 9, list the steps to complete Plan B.
    *Ex:* Plan B Steps for *Get professional help for my emotions*:
    ✓ Call the Veterans' Administration or my health insurance company.
    ✓ Make an appointment for the soonest date possible and keep it.

    Your Plan B
    ✓ _____
    ✓ _____
    ✓ _____
    ✓ _____
    ✓ _____
    ✓ _____

12. Take the steps, then review whether and how they worked; if necessary, define new solution ideas and steps.
    _____
    _____
    _____
    _____
    _____

13. Regardless of the outcomes, whether or not the problem was totally resolved, what did you learn about your attitudes, abilities and the feasibility of your ideas?
    _____
    _____
    _____
    _____
    _____

*(Continued)*

INSIGHT AND EMPOWERMENT

## Problems Can Be Opportunities *(Continued)*

14. Think about a current problem; describe what you did to help remedy or decrease it, or a similar problem, in the past, (even if it helped only a little bit).
    _____
    _____
    _____
    _____
    _____

15. What have you been doing to keep the problem from worsening?
    _____
    _____
    _____
    _____
    _____

16. How can you do more of what works or do it better?
    _____
    _____
    _____
    _____
    _____

17. Share what you are doing or productive actions you can take to fulfill yourself in each area:
    - ✓ Survival _____
    - ✓ Love and Belonging _____
    - ✓ Power _____
    - ✓ Freedom _____
    - ✓ Fun _____

18. Some destructive habits are criticizing, blaming, complaining, nagging, threatening, punishing, and bribing or rewarding to control. How have you hurt yourself and others by doing any or all of these?
    _____
    _____
    _____
    _____

19. Constructive habits include supporting, encouraging, listening, accepting, trusting, respecting, and negotiating differences. Share how you are using, or will implement, these in your most important relationship(s):
    _____
    _____
    _____
    _____

20. How will your relationships and mood improve by practicing constructive habits?
    _____
    _____
    _____

# Art Activities Facilitators Guide

## Measureable Behavioral Goals

**For veterans who will depict any or all of these scenarios ...**
- A serene location, plus inner peace.
- Themselves larger than their enemies and bravely facing challenges.
- People, experiences, attributes, and possibilities for which they are thankful.
- Their worst and best of times, lessons learned and peak experiences.
- Their fears outside; their strengths, comforts and coping skills; their inside safety zones.
- They will also apply related quotes to their pictures and their lives.

## This Guide is for the following separate art exercises:
- I – A Peaceful Place
- II – A Winning Warrior
- III – Gratitude
- IV – Pits and Peaks
- V – Safety Zones

## Introduction
1. Provide 8½ x 11 paper or larger; consider tan or white butcher paper, an easel paper roll, the back of wrapping paper; pencils, crayons, paints, colored marker pens. Big paper and many supplies promote creativity.
2. Before the session read and retain this guide and the reproducible pages.
3. Ideally, the activities will be used on different days; the reproducible pages have lines for cutting out and photocopying the topic you wish to use for each session.
4. Alternatively, you may choose to distribute all reproducible pages; participants select different topics depending on their preferences, needs or focus issues.

## Activity
1. Distribute the cut out portion of the reproducible page(s) you choose to use.
2. Take turns reading aloud the Education portion.
3. Explain that artistic talent is irrelevant; the process of expression is important.
4. Ask them to stay silent during the drawing and focus on their own work.
5. When all are done, encourage them to show and describe about their projects.

## Conclusion
- Ask them to share their responses to the quotation(s).

Note: There are no Interactive Variations suggested for these very introspective art activities.

# Art Activities

## I – A Peaceful Place

**Education**

- You can be calm in chaos by re-experiencing a peaceful place: the beach, mountains, forest, wherever soothes your senses.
- Colors, temperatures, sights, sounds, fragrances, and feeling the breeze or sand, contribute to the atmosphere.
- Imagine your place at any time, anywhere, to focus your mind and relax.

**Insight and Empowerment**

1. Draw the most tranquil place you have ever been; use colors that calm you.
2. On the other side of your drawing, or separate page, depict your inner peace.
3. You may instead, or in addition to the above drawings, illustrate this quote by Mahatma Gandhi:

*Each one of us has to find his peace from within.*
*And peace to be real must be unaffected by outside circumstances.*

4. Apply the quotation to you and elaborate on your drawings in writing.

## II – A Winning Warrior

**Education**

- You are back from war but may be fighting different foes.
- They may loom large; you may feel dwarfed; you can adopt a winning mind-set.
- Visualize yourself fighting bravely to diminish and defeat your demons.

**Insight and Empowerment**

1. Draw yourself larger than your enemies, facing current challenges bravely.
2. Depict smaller enemies: people and situations that seemingly threaten you.
3. You may prefer a cartoon with captions showing your positive self-talk.
4. You may instead, or in addition to the above drawing, illustrate this quote by Sun-Tzu:

*Victorious warriors win first and then go to war,*
*while defeated warriors go to war first and then seek to win.*

5. Apply the quotation to you and elaborate on your drawings in writing.

# Art Activities

## III – Gratitude

**Education**

- Gratitude helps focus on positives versus dwelling on the destruction of war.
- Thankfulness helps reduce stress and lift mood.

**Insight and Empowerment**

1. Draw in collage form or in any way you wish, depicting everything and everyone you are thankful for.
2. Add
   - Difficult experiences that led to a stronger you.
   - Your attributes.
   - Positive outcomes you envision for your future.
3. You may instead, or in addition to the above drawing, illustrate this quote by Kak Sri:

*Gratitude is an art of painting adversity into a lovely picture.*

4. Apply the quotation to you and elaborate on your drawing in writing.

## IV – Pits and Peaks

**Education**

- Have you been in the pits, or in the trenches?
- Tragedies and low points happen, particularly in war and its aftermath.
- Peak experiences exhilarate in the midst of a crisis, or at other times and places.
- Peak experiences are external or internal triumphs.
- Peak experiences are light bulb moments of insight, foresight and hindsight.

**Insight and Empowerment**

1. At the bottom left of the paper, draw your worst of times.
2. On the right side of the page, draw a big mountain.
3. On the mountain, draw your best of times; fun, learning, making it to the summit.
4. At its peak, draw your greatest act, attribute, idea, and future expectations.
5. You may instead, or in addition to the above drawing, illustrate this quote by Nelson Mandela:

*There is no easy walk to freedom anywhere, and many of us will have to pass through the shadow of death again and again before we reach the mountaintop of our desires.*

6. Apply the quotation to you and elaborate on your drawing in writing.

# Art Activities

## V – Safety Zones

### Education

- Wartime safety zones include foxholes, mine resistant ambush protected (MRAP) vehicles, fortified tents, underground bunkers and bomb shelters.
- You may be out of the war zone but still tormented by memories, dreams, flashbacks, sights, fears, sounds, smells, thoughts and feelings.
- You have inner strengths, external resources and coping skills to protect you.

### Insight and Empowerment

1. Use pictures, symbols, cartoons, and/or colors in collage form, or in other ways.
2. Outline your tent, vehicle, shelter or other safety zone.
3. Outside, draw everything that scares you.
4. Inside, draw you, with everything that
   - Saves
   - Strengthens
   - Calms
   - Helps you cope
   - Gives you hope

5. You may instead, or in addition to the above drawing, illustrate one or both quotes:

   *To live with Fear and not be afraid is the final test of maturity.*
   ~ Edward Weeks

   *You cannot always control what goes on outside,*
   *but you can always control what goes on inside.*
   ~ Dr. Wayne Dyer

6. Apply the quotations to you and elaborate on your drawings in writing.

# The Mighty Pen Facilitator's Guide

## Measurable Behavioral Objectives

**Veterans will ...**
- State reasons they enlisted and the degree to which expectations were met.
- Identify military-related changes in themselves and relationships.
- Identify lessons learned, and who and how they can now teach or inspire.
- Describe their buddies, memories and plans to stay connected or to memorialize.
- Describe the place they served and its people; whether to return and why.
- Elaborate on song lyrics or use them as starters and write their own lines.
- Consider a wrong they hoped to right or other belief; decide if *the pen is mightier than the sword*, why, and empower their pens by promoting their cause.
- Analyze a quote about advancing in a different direction versus retreating.
- Read a quote about success and share how they are bouncing back.
- Write letters of advice to persons pondering service or new service members.
- Write about anything: dreams; what angers, dismays, delights or inspires them.

## Introduction

1. Before the session begins, read this guide and the reproducible pages.
2. Decide whether to distribute the list of topics for self-selection, or whether you will assign a different topic on different days.
3. Photocopy the reproducible pages but retain them until after the introduction; or make only one copy for yourself and plan to introduce a single topic only.
4. Write the word *Journaling* on the board and ask if any have written in diaries or journals and how it helped them.
5. Explain they will be writing on issues near and dear to their hearts.

## Activity

1. Reinforce that editing for spelling and grammar come later; emphasize the importance of process and uncensored content.
2. Distribute the reproducible pages, take turns reading aloud the Education portion, and direct group members to select one of the Insight and Assessment topics to write about.
3. If you choose one of the topics, read the Education portion to participants and write the related text onto the board; do not share the list; use for future sessions.
4. Allow time to complete the written Insight and Empowerment exercise.
5. Encourage group members to share their work if they wish.

## Conclusion

- Ask participants share benefits from writing and ways they will continue journaling.

## Interactive Variation

- Journaling is introspective; sharing segments of one's writing is interactive and should not be required.

EDUCATION & INSIGHT AND EMPOWERMENT

# The Mighty Pen

## Education

Writing for self-understanding and growth has nothing to do with spelling, grammar or beautiful penmanship. It is getting your thoughts on paper, for analysis and clarification. Journaling releases emotions, improves mood, increases resilience, and helps healing.

Your work is for your eyes only; don't clean it up; go with the flow; no censorship. The process matters. You may choose to share, shred, or lock up your work.

- Select any of the topics below or make up your own.
- Set aside quiet time and space to write daily.
- Just do it, even if you don't feel inspired.
- The topics below are starters; after a while ideas will pop into your head.

## Insight and Empowerment

1. How did you happen to enlist? Share your initial ideas, and reasons. Discuss how your military experience fell short, met or exceeded your expectations.

2. How have your military experiences changed you, your partner, family, relationships, career plans and other aspects of your life? How have your beliefs, values and faith changed? What changes would you now like to make in yourself, your life and relationships?

3. Share thoughts or memories of a commander, instructor, or superior in the military who taught you valuable lessons. What did you learn, and how did it help you in the service? How does this learning apply to civilian life? Additionally, share thoughts about a family member, teacher, coach, or other person who taught you. What did you learn? Who can you now inspire and how?

4. Write about a poor role model. What did this person do that you will never do? In what ways will you not treat others? How are you overcoming the impact this person had on your life?

5. Share about one or a few best buddies: How did you become friends? What are your happiest and saddest memories about them? What made your relationship special compared to civilian friendships? How do you plan to stay connected? If they have passed, how will you keep their memory alive?

6. Share memories or thoughts about the place you were stationed, the sights, sounds, smells, types of food you ate, and living conditions. How did the people, their customs and culture affect you? Describe the beautiful and ugly memories. How do you feel about returning to visit this place?

7. What songs were popular during your service? Write or paraphrase their lyrics. How do they affect you? Think about other favorite songs, quote a few lines, then create your own endings.

*(Continued on the next page)*

## INSIGHT AND EMPOWERMENT

# The Mighty Pen *(Continued)*

8. Consider Edward Bulwer-Lytton's words:

    ***The pen is mightier than the sword.***

    - Describe why you agree or disagree.
    - How or when did you potentially risk your life for a cause, to right a wrong?
    - Make your pen mighty: promote your ideas about social justice, your pet peeve, improving the armed services, regulations or laws you would like to institute or change, or other passionate beliefs.

9. Consider the words of General Douglas MacArthur:

    ***We are not retreating – we are advancing in another direction.***

    - How are you not hiding or running from a problem at this time?
    - How are you progressing in a new direction?
    - What are or will be your victories?

10. Consider the words of George S. Patton:

    ***Success is how high you bounce when you hit bottom.***

    - Describe what it means when you hit bottom.
    - Identify ways you are bouncing back and how you plan to reach new heights.

11. Write a letter of advice to a young person who is considering enlisting; include pros and cons. Or, write to a person who has enlisted; give advice about aspects you consider important (combat? training? relationships? returning home? etc.)

12. Write about any topic in any way you wish.
    - What is on your mind today?
    - What is in your nightmares or dreams?
    - What do you daydream about?
    - What angers, dismays, delights or inspires you?
    - How do you react to nature, sun and/or storms?

COPING SKILLS

# Express Yourself Facilitator's Guide

## Measurable Behavioral Objectives

**Veterans will ...**
- Read about and be referred to music, dance, drama, poetry and fiction writing resources for veterans.
- Describe a time, place, situation, memories and music that were meaningful.
- Share preferences and plans for listening, singing or playing music.
- Discuss mixing music with dance, or watching, coaching or playing sports to enthuse and energize.
- Describe a story or play with at least eleven components, (plot, characters, etc.).
- Write a poem about a subject of personal importance.
- Discuss the most important books they have read, favorite authors and preferred types of literature.
- Begin creating themselves by sharing five aspects of an autobiography.
- Have the opportunity to actually sing, play an instrument, listen to music, compose lyrics, write or act in a play, as part of their group experience; collaborate with peers; form clubs to read and discuss their chosen books.

## Introduction

1. Before the session begins, read this guide and the reproducible pages.
2. Decide whether you wish to add one of the interactive activities to a session before or after this activity.
3. Photocopy the reproducible pages but retain them until after the introduction.
4. Write *Creativity* on the board and ask participants to brainstorm ways people are creative.
5. Explain that they will be exposed to types of expressive therapy.

## Activity

1. Distribute the reproducible pages.
2. Take turns reading the Education portion aloud.
3. Allow time to complete the written Insight and Empowerment questions.
4. Encourage participants to share their responses to question numbers 1-3, and number 6.

## Conclusion

- Encourage participants to share about their choice of a story or play (number 4), poem (number 5) or autobiography (number 7).

## Interactive Enrichment Activities

- In addition to completing the preceding exercises, consider the following and use your imagination for other ideas:
- Use a karaoke machine, microphone and music for a song fest.
- Bring printed lyrics and sing A Capella or along with a CD or video.
- Encourage people to bring in and play instruments for the group.
- Have a dance along to a video or teach each other dance steps.
- Start book clubs: small sub-groups with similar preferences read and discuss a chapter a week from their chosen book.
- Pairs or teams collaborate on a song, poem or play; then read lyrics or poems to others, perform their plays, or direct others to act in their plays.

© 2013 WHOLE PERSON ASSOCIATES, 101 WEST 2ND ST., SUITE 203, DULUTH MN 55802 ▪ 800-247-6789

EDUCATION

# Express Yourself

**For all expressive exercises, focus on getting your thoughts and feelings out; gather tools - pen, paper, paint, canvas, etc. There is no right or wrong way. Put perfection and professionalism aside.**

## Music

Veterans have been soothed with music since World War I; Veterans Administration (VA) Hospitals used music therapy during both World Wars and thereafter.

- Music activates memories, feelings and pleasure centers in the brain.
- Music decreases fear and anxiety, helping veterans to talk about upsetting events.
- Low pitched and slower songs are more soothing than high pitched voices and instruments.
- Melodies may lull you to sleep.
- Some songs or music helpful to soldiers suffering from trauma are Amazing Grace, Oh Danny Boy, Memory, Beethoven's 9th Symphony, The Marines' Hymn; etc.
- Be open to different types of music and perhaps you'll find new favorites.
- The music of your youth may work for you if those were happy times; be sure your selections don't trigger drug or alcohol associations or cravings.
- The songs popular during your service may help or hurt; you decide.
- Consider visiting senior centers and provide musical entertainment and sing-alongs.

## Movement and Dance

Dancing gets you out of the doldrums. It is used in VA Hospitals; veterans speak with their bodies what they cannot put into words.

- Just as with exercise or yoga, external movement affects internal emotions.
- Dancing affects your well-being, brightens your mood.
- Avoid self-criticism or comparison with others.
- You are not in a contest; you're in it for fun.
- Whether you like country western, ballroom, ethnic, or hip hop, just dance!

## Creative Writing

Unlike journaling, (your informal personal essay or diary), creative writing produces a story, commentary, play or poem, or poses a research idea. Remember process matters more than product; forget perfect grammar or form.

- Poetry need not rhyme.
- Publication is possible but should not be the driving force.
- Use your imagination: storytelling, true to life characters, dilemmas, decisions matter.
- Your own life and experiences are food for thought.
- You can be wild and crazy and use people, places and things totally new to you.
- Try writing rap or romantic songs, be upbeat or sentimental. Choices are endless.

## Bibliotherapy

Reading and relating to books, prose, poetry, or audio tapes of books helps you explore emotions and ideas.

- Decide the type of books you like, fiction, non-fiction, science fiction, war stories, murder mysteries, romance, westerns, poetry, self-help books and workbooks, etc.
- Check libraries, on-line options, half-price or swap bookstores, coffee house book stores.
- Consider book or library clubs where you read all or portions of a book and meet for discussion.

INSIGHT AND EMPOWERMENT

# Express Yourself

1. Share a time when a song or instrumental composition was meaningful: where were you, with whom? Name the songs; describe the memories. Will it help or hurt to hear that music today? Why and how?

2. If you like music, how can you incorporate it into your life? In addition to listening, would you like to sing or play an instrument? Might you join a choir at your house of worship or in your community? Take a college or adult music education class? Use local karaoke opportunities? Check online for instruction and other options especially for veterans. Share your preferences and plans:

3. Dancing might accompany listening to your favorite music at home; additionally lessons and resources especially for veterans are available. Sports can excite and energize whether you are watching, coaching or playing. Describe your favorite types of dance or sports and how you will incorporate them into your life.

4. Share ideas about a short story, novel, epic poem, magazine article or play. Describe the following:
    a. Setting, time and location. _____
    b. Plot or storyline. _____
    c. Main characters. _____
    d. Conflicts and challenges. _____
    e. What do the characters discover about themselves and each other? _____
    f. What dilemmas and decisions do they face? _____
    g. What secrets do they reveal? _____
    h. Describe a turning point when the main characters accept or reject what they thought. _____
    i. Imagine the drama. _____
    j. Describe the most exciting event. _____
    k. Describe how it might, or might not be resolved. _____

5. Try your hand at a poem. Write about something near and dear, an emotion, an incident, a person, a place, patriotism, the past, the present, the future, combat, homecoming, life, liberty, trauma, healing, etc. Go with the flow of your heart and soul. Do not edit or try to perfect a poem. Penetrate the paper with your ideas.

6. Share thoughts about your favorite types of books, titles, authors, themes and topics. What book made the biggest impression on you and how? What would you like to read within the next six months and why?

7. ***But if you have nothing at all to create, then perhaps create yourself.*** ~Carl Gustav Jung
Consider writing your autobiography; tell it like it is or fictionalize the story and recreate yourself: give yourself the qualities you admire; describe doing what you've always wanted to do; overcome obstacles; reach for the stars. Try viewing past trauma as growth opportunity and see yourself strengthened; make your future happen as you wish. Share at least five aspects of your acknowledged self.

# Relationships

*"When we seek to discover the best in others,
we somehow bring out the best in ourselves."*

~ William Arthur Ward

**Veterans will identify** risks for infidelity among military couples and how they might improve their current or future relationships. They will learn ways to help survive a break-up and to help their children adapt to single parent homes. Participants will focus on strength from adversity, finding support systems and engaging in self-renewal.

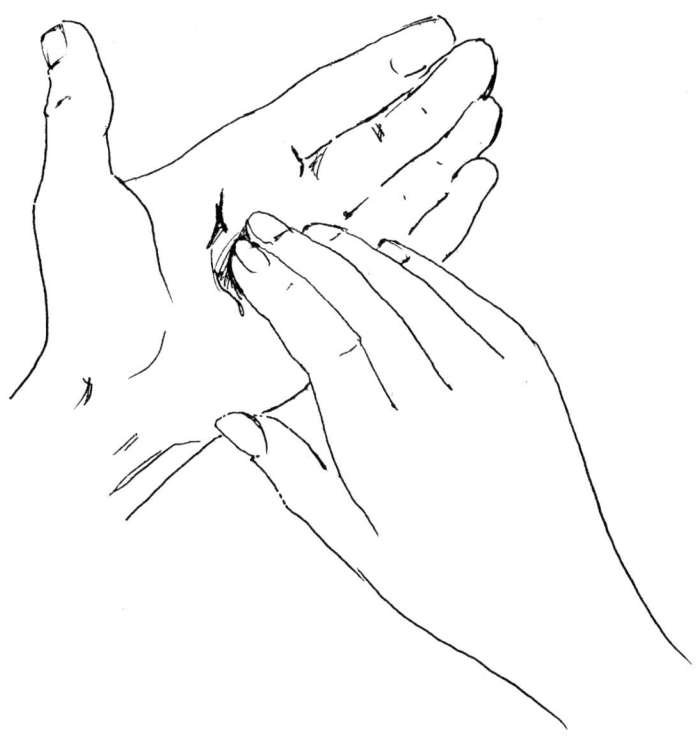

VETERANS: SURVIVING AND THRIVING AFTER TRAUMA

# Infidelity and Introspection Facilitator's Guide

## Measurable Behavioral Objectives

**Veterans will …**
- Rate their relationship regarding risks for infidelity related to military couples.
- Identify contributing factors within and outside of themselves.
- Seek counsel from a therapist or spiritual advisor, if needed.
- Describe their feelings whether they were betrayed or strayed.
- Identify dangerous responses to avoid.
- State how they might grow from this crisis.
- Identify people and coping skills to help them through the crisis of divorce or reconciliation.
- List their major needs or expectations from a relationship.
- Identify, with hindsight, what they might have done differently.

## Introduction

1. Before the session begins, read this guide and the reproducible pages.
2. Decide on one of the interactive activities or the traditional approach (below).
3. Photocopy the reproducible pages but retain them until after the introduction.
4. Write the word *Infidelity* on the board and ask why affairs might occur among military couples.
5. A volunteer lists their ideas on the board.
6. Explain this activity is the *tip of the iceberg* in a troubled marriage; they will benefit from professional counseling.

## Activity

1. Distribute the reproducible pages.
2. Take turns reading the Education and Assessment portion aloud.
3. Encourage participants to check the applicable boxes.
4. Allow time to complete the written Insight and Empowerment questions.
5. Encourage group members to share their responses.

## Conclusion

- Encourage a discussion regarding military situations that may lead to infidelity, and what changes in policies and procedures might better promote committed relationships.

## Interactive Variations

- Ask participants to take turns reading the Insight and Empowerment questions aloud and answering orally.
- Ask them to pair up with peers, read the questions to each other, record their partner's responses, then share with the group if they wish.

EDUCATION AND ASSESSMENT & INSIGHT AND EMPOWERMENT

# Infidelity and Introspection

## Education and Assessment

**Infidelity among military couples has many possible reasons. Check the boxes for your risk factors.**
- ❏ Drinking or drugs diminish inhibitions in war zones or at home.
- ❏ The thought of imminent death may cause you to seize the moment.
- ❏ Multiple deployments and distances contribute to loneliness and secrecy.
- ❏ Adventurous affairs decrease the drudgery of combat or homebound duties.
- ❏ Proximity of buddies, or best friends stateside, promotes blossoming into lovers.
- ❏ Getting even occurs when people think their partner is cheating.
- ❏ Emotional conditions may diminish libido; partners who feel rejected may seek sex elsewhere.
- ❏ Emotionally disturbed, detached or angry partners may stray.

Additional considerations:
- Poor communication, unmet needs, unequal sharing of responsibilities for children, chores or finances.
- Most affairs do not become permanent; they fizzle out on their own or due to interventions by betrayed partners; but separation or divorce may result.
- Expect a roller-coaster of love-hate feelings; get immediate help if you feel like harming yourself or others.
- Unresolved sexual, emotional or addiction issues can be helped.
- Religious and other spiritual counselors will help.
- Military legal assistance is available if divorce is planned.
- If you are thinking about suicide, with a plan and a means to carry it out, call 911 or your local Emergency Services number, the National Suicide Prevention Lifeline/Veteran's Crisis Line.1-800-273-8255 (TALK), or go to your nearest hospital Emergency Room.

## Insight and Empowerment

Introspection is the detailed examination of your own thoughts, feelings and motives.

**If you strayed or have been betrayed:**

1. Take time out to cry, breathe, meditate and deliberate. Describe your initial thoughts and feelings about the infidelity.

2. Blaming yourself, your spouse, or the other person is unproductive. Honestly explore any contribution you might have made to the situation.

3. Objectively consider the circumstances: What other factors contributed to the affair: many deployments, addictions, emotional problems or history of being sexually abused, etc.?

4. If you decide on divorce or reconciliation, who, and what skills, will help you through the crisis?

5. Avoid dangerous behaviors like drinking, drugging, driving recklessly, promiscuity or aggressive acts in response to relationship problems. What specifically do you need to avoid?

6. In what ways have you grown or might you grow from this crisis?

7. The second time around (with this partner or in a future relationship), what will be your three major needs or expectations?

8. With the wisdom of *Monday morning quarterbacking*, what might you have done differently?

# Surviving a Breakup Facilitator's Guide

## Measurable Behavioral Objectives

**Veterans will ...**
- Identify strains on military relationships and resources for marital counseling.
- Identify ways to help their children survive parental separation.
- Describe their experiences of a breakup or divorce.
- Discuss anger, forgiveness and advantages of being single in their situations.
- Avoid rebound relationships, but decide qualities they seek in a future partner.
- Share lessons learned and describe their personal renewal plan.
- Practice positive self-talk regarding strength, thriving and facing challenges.
- State how helping others or productive activity helps them recover.
- Apply inspirational quotes regarding transformation, love and moving forward in their lives.

## Introduction

1. Before the session begins, read this guide and the reproducible pages.
2. Decide on one of the interactive activities or the traditional approach (below).
3. Photocopy the reproducible pages but retain them until after the introduction.
4. Ask group members to brainstorm reasons for military divorces.
5. A volunteer lists reasons on the board.
6. Explian there are many resources to assist in a crisis, and for counseling or divorce recovery.

## Activity

1. Distribute the reproducible pages.
2. Take turns reading aloud the Education and Assessment portion.
3. Encourage participants to check the applicable boxes as they read.
4. Allow time to complete the written Insight and Empowerment questions.
5. Encourage participants to share their answers through number 10.

## Conclusion

- Encourage group members to analyze and apply the quotations to their lives (numbers 11-14).

## Interactive Variations

- Ask participants to take turns reading the Insight and Empowerment questions aloud and answering them orally, with the group if they wish.
- Ask participants to pair up with peers, read the questions to each other, record their partner's responses, then share with the group if they wish.

EDUCATION AND ASSESSMENT

# Surviving a Breakup

**Military relationships, in which one or both partners are veterans, are often strained. Multiple deployments and long distances and durations apart make some partners feel like strangers.**

- Sharing feelings versus building up resentments, demonstrating willingness to work on issues versus a quick fix, and agreeing to counseling for emotional, addiction and relationship problems may help.

- Often, one partner hopes to salvage the union and the other wants out. If divorce is inevitable, the military offers assistance; see websites and resources pages 159–163. Veterans facing separation and divorce will find legal and financial information.

- If you are thinking about suicide, with a plan and a means to carry it out, call 911 or your local Emergency Services number, the National Suicide Prevention Lifeline/Veteran's Crisis Line 1-800-273-8255 (TALK), or go to your nearest hospital Emergency Room.

- Saving a life is crucial, regardless of whether the marriage can be saved.

## The Kids

Check the boxes that are helpful in your situation:

- ❏ Prioritize your children's emotional and financial needs. Tell them as much in advance as possible, encourage them to express their feelings, and assure them the separation is not their fault. Allow them to continue supportive family ties with the other parent's relatives. Divorce may be a relief for them if there was extreme conflict, or it may be a shock with devastating consequences.

- ❏ Plan visitation or joint custody until terms of the divorce are final. Do not interrogate kids upon return from visits. Do not bad mouth your spouse to the children or make them messengers or marriage counselors; they love both parents who both love them.

- ❏ Education and counseling are available for effective co-parenting. Children do survive divorced upbringing, especially when both parents are on the same page regarding rules and discipline. Children can thrive in loving single or remarried parents' homes.

- ❏ Marriage and family therapists, school counselors, religious and spiritual guides will be helpful.

- ❏ Be involved in your children's activities and try not to disrupt their routines. Seek out a support network for them in sports or other activities that are within your scope for cost, time, transportation, etc.

- ❏ Be an example for your kids. Show how to handle disappointments or crises with kindness, faith and hope; there is life after divorce for you and the children.

- ❏ You or the children may be eligible for some social service assistance funds, child care, decreased utility costs, or other benefits. Check with your County Department of Public Social Services and your utility companies. Housing assistance and food stamps may be available, depending on income.

## INSIGHT AND EMPOWERMENT
# Surviving a Breakup

1. Expect to go through the process of denial, anger, grief and acceptance. Describe your experiences with
   a. Denial _____
   b. Anger _____
   c. Grief _____
   d. Acceptance _____

2. Continue and strengthen ties with friends and family; or make new friends if your couples friends shun you; divorce support groups and religious, spiritual and other organizations can help. Surround yourself with non-judgmental, optimistic people. List at least three sources for your emotional support:
   _____
   _____

3. Express your anger and feelings to a friend or therapist; do not dwell on revenge. Who is your sounding board and what thoughts, feelings and issues do you plan to discuss? If it is a friend, keep it at five to fifteen minutes and then go on with different discussions, including asking about the other person.
   _____
   _____

4. Try to avoid blame. Relationships end; people move on. Discuss how you are forgiving others or yourself:
   _____
   _____

5. Decide it is acceptable to be single for now. What are three advantages of your current situation?
   _____
   _____

6. Avoid a rapid rebound affair; a replacement romance rarely lasts. The time frame for starting to date is different for each person. When you enter a relationship, remember that your ex is the children's other parent, and if they remain involved, discuss child-rearing and finances with the other parent, versus expecting the new person to usurp the other parent's role. What three qualities are crucial for a person you bring into your and your children's lives?
   _____
   _____

7. What three most important lessons have you learned from your relationship and the break-up?
   _____
   _____

8. Rather than dwelling on the end of your partnership, focus on a new beginning for yourself. What new information will benefit you or your career via online research, a class, a training program, or other method? Describe your personal renewal plan:
   _____
   _____

INSIGHT AND EMPOWERMENT

# Surviving a Breakup *(Continued)*

9. Positive self-talk is imperative. Write three statements regarding
   a. Strength you gained from adversity:_____
   b. Your current surviving and thriving strategies:_____
   c. Your newest challenge: _____

10. Helping others helps you. Volunteer at a shelter, food bank, or animal rescue; engage in social reform or political action work, help at your children's schools or activities, support others going through breakups. If you are in school or working, plus have children to care for, you may be scheduled *to the max*. What is your *passion* or *pet project* and how will you fit that one activity or challenge into your schedule?
   _____

11. How does this Richard Bach quote describe you?

    ***What the caterpillar calls the end of the world, the master calls the butterfly.***

    _____
    _____
    _____
    _____

12. Agree, disagree, and elaborate your thoughts on this Alfred Lord Tennyson quote:

    ***Tis better to have loved and lost than never to have loved at all.***

    _____
    _____
    _____
    _____

13. Apply to your life this Albert Einstein quote:

    ***Life is like riding a bicycle. To keep your balance, you must keep moving.***

    _____
    _____
    _____
    _____

14. Describe your paralysis prevention plan suggested by Florence Nightingale:

    ***The choice is pain or paralysis.***

    _____
    _____
    _____
    _____

# Rebounding

*"Start by doing what's necessary; then do what's possible; and suddenly you are doing the impossible."*

~ St. Francis of Assisi

**V**ETERANS WILL LEARN TO IDENTIFY ways to face and heal from physical and psychological wounds of war. They will analyze their stereotypes regarding people with disabilities and discover resources, new roles and values. They will learn that their disability need not define them. They will explore resources for pain management and physical well-being. They will consider ways to set and work toward high goals of wellness intellectually, physically, emotionally, socially, spiritually and vocationally.

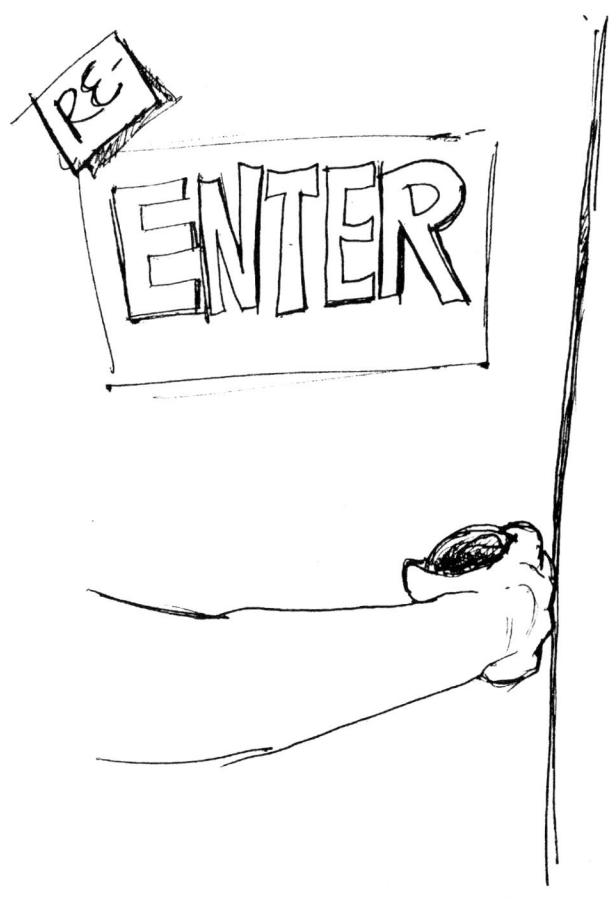

# Broken Bodies Facilitator's Guide

## Measurable Behavioral Objectives

**Veterans will ...**
- Rate themselves regarding common responses to disfigurements or impairments.
- Read about services available to veterans and families.
- Compare their prior perceptions of people with disabilities to their current views.
- State negative and positive prior traits that impede or promote recovery.
- Identify new traits that help them adapt.
- Redefine roles, incorporating new ways to fulfill them.
- Learn to read information about medications.
- Rate themselves regarding non-medicinal pain management techniques.
- Acknowledge they must check with their physician regarding any interventions.
- Rate themselves regarding options for improved appearance and mobility.
- Complete exercises promoting cognitive changes and addressing physical, emotional, intellectual, social, spiritual and vocational aspects of recovery.
- Apply quotations to their abilities and futures.

## Introduction

1. Before the session begins, read this guide and the reproducible pages.
2. Decide on one of the interactive variations or the traditional approach (below).
3. Photocopy the reproducible pages but retain them until after the introduction.
4. Ask, *"After an injury, when does rehabilitation begin?"* Elicit that recovery and rehabilitation begin the first day.
5. Ask each person to share personal progress, physical and psychological, since the day of injury.

## Activity

1. Distribute the reproducible pages.
2. Take turns reading the Education and Assessment portion aloud.
3. Encourage participants to check the applicable boxes.
4. Allow time to complete the written Insight and Empowerment questions.
5. Encourage them to share their responses through number 10.

## Conclusion

- Encourage participants to share their responses to the quotations (numbers 11-14).

## Interactive Variations

- Ask participants to take turns reading the Insight and Empowerment questions aloud and answering orally.
- Ask them to pair up with peers, read the questions to each other, record their partner's responses, then share with the group if they wish.

EDUCATION AND ASSESSMENT

# Broken Bodies

*"Oh no! Not me! How will I survive?"*

Broken bodies bring broken hearts. Intimate relationships, friendships, family, finances and faith are shaken.

Combat wounds often result in a physical or mental impairment that substantially limits one or more major life activities.

**Check boxes below that apply to your situation:**

- ❏ I feel lonely or abandoned.
- ❏ I am living in low-cost or special housing with an associated stigma.
- ❏ I see myself as "less than" because of physical limits, inability to walk or work.
- ❏ People act uncomfortable around me.
- ❏ I am frustrated by delays in financial, medical or rehabilitation assistance.
- ❏ I am experiencing shock, anger, resentment, grief and loss regarding bodily functions.
- ❏ I have work, financial, and relationship problems.
- ❏ I am experiencing pain; low energy.
- ❏ I am experiencing changes in eating; sleeping.
- ❏ I am noticing changes in my sexual life.
- ❏ My self-image has changed; I am hiding from the public; I am embarrassed.
- ❏ I feel that some of my independence is gone.

Numerous resources for veterans are available. See the Resources chapter and know that your Department of Veterans Affairs has information and services regarding the following, plus other benefits: Disability Compensation, Health Care and Life Insurance Benefits, Automobile Allowance and help with adaptive devices, Vocational Rehabilitation, Employment, Home Modification; see **http://www.va.gov** and the Resource Section in this book, pages 159–163.

Military branches have Wounded Warrior programs which help with health, recreation, adaptive bicycles and other sports needs; prostheses; backpacks with supplies for hospital stays; education and training; family retreats and support; and connections to other wounded veterans.

**If you have a disability, remember:**

- Despite the impairment, you remain more like others and like your old self, than different.
- You bring your abilities, limitations, goals and personality to the situation.
- You are not a disabled person, but a person with a disability.
- Your disability does not define you!
- You are still YOU!

## INSIGHT AND EMPOWERMENT
# Broken Bodies

**Effects of Stereotypes**

1. Describe at least five impressions you had of people in wheel chairs or with other disabilities or facial disfigurements before you got hurt:

2. How is your view of yourself similar to your prior stereotype?

3. In what ways is your self-concept different from your prior stereotype?

4. Describe three of your prior positive traits and how they are helping you to cope:

5. Describe three of your prior negative traits and how they handicap your progress:

6. Describe three new positive traits you developed since the injury and how they are helping you to adapt:

**Redefining Roles**

Regarding roles, you may have some limitations. Focus on what you can do; redefine your values regarding what makes a good partner, parent, patriot, worker, etc.

| Role | Old Values | Old Abilities | New Values | New Abilities |
|---|---|---|---|---|
| Example: Parent | Playing sports with kids shows love. | Play softball, tennis; able to run, throw and hit balls. | Showing interest in their sports shows love. | Attend their games; do lifeguard supervised water activities with them. |
| Example: Lover | Sexual acts show love. | Performance. | Kindness, caring, and communication show love. | Listen, share feelings, show emotional, physical and sexual affection. |
| | | | | |
| | | | | |
| | | | | |
| | | | | |
| | | | | |

INSIGHT AND EMPOWERMENT

# Major Life Activities

Quality of life includes physical, emotional, intellectual, social, spiritual and vocational functioning.

Physical problems after an injury include phantom limb or other pain and your doctor may order prescriptions or over the counter medications.

Always check with your doctor and read labels about interactions, precautions and side-effects.

Non-medicinal pain management is important and empowering.

Check boxes regarding interventions you use or will try with your physician's approval:
- ❏ Heat or cold: be sure to limit the time and control the temperature.
- ❏ Mild exercise, massage therapy, over-the-counter patches and liniments.
- ❏ Acupuncture: needles inserted at strategic points by an acupuncturist.
- ❏ Aromatherapy: using pleasant scents to relax and lift mood.
- ❏ Biofeedback: machine or your pulse show tenseness; lower pulse and relax.
- ❏ Breathing: practice blowing big bubbles; use that technique when in pain.
- ❏ Distractions: TV, animals, art, music, cards, games, books.
- ❏ Guided imagery: tapes or self talk, to guide you to experience peaceful places with all senses.
- ❏ Humor: watch funny movies and TV; read jokes; have a sense of humor.

**For your emotional health, a positive attitude and active participation in therapy are essential.**

1. Change two negative ideas about your injury to positive but realistic thoughts: See examples below.
   ***Example*** – Negative: *People will be repulsed by my appearance.*
   Positive: *I'll improve what I can; I'll seek people who value my internal qualities.*
   ***Example*** – Negative: *I'm imprisoned in my wheelchair.*
   Positive: *I can play wheelchair basketball and race; most places are wheelchair accessible.*

Negative: _____
Positive: _____

Negative: _____
Positive: _____

Negative: _____
Positive: _____

Negative: _____
Positive: _____

Negative: _____
Positive: _____

*(Continued on the next page)*

## INSIGHT AND EMPOWERMENT

# Major Life Activities *(continued)*

2. Your disability is not your identity. Complete the sentences below about aspects of you unaffected or improved by your injury:
   a. I think ... _____
   b. I believe ... _____
   c. I am ... _____
   d. I love ... _____
   e. I will ... _____

3. For enhancing your intellectual health, you need stimulation such as reading, puzzles, crosswords, Sudoku, writing, and other activities. What will you do daily for mental fitness?
   _____
   _____

4. For your intellectual health and to support your well-being, you need knowledge about your physical condition, medications, and treatment options. How will or do you use the Internet, publications, videos, and support groups to arm you with knowledge?
   _____
   _____

5. For your social life, you need to be loved and to belong to a family or group of friends. Some people blame their disabilities for social disconnections, but do things to alienate others. Share examples of times you might have done the following:
   a. Displaced anger onto a loved one: _____
   b. Acted too independent, refused needed help: _____
   c. Acted too needy: _____

6. In your social life, you need people who understand, look beyond a scar or missing limb, and have similar interests. Veteran and other support groups are helpful if they focus on recovery; hobbies, classes, clubs, religious or spiritual activities, and online communities help. Where and how might you find friends or a dating partner?
   _____
   _____

7. For your spiritual life, you need hope and faith to get through tough times and look forward to the future. Inspirational literature, art, music, poetry, nature and nurturing people are external sources. Faith in self or a Higher Power, perseverance, boldness, motivation, and other internal qualities will sustain you.
   a. Share three sources of external inspiration: _____
   b. Share three of your inner strengths: _____

8. In your vocational life, you may be able to do a prior patriotic duty or civilian job with modifications or you may need re-training. Remember, one's job title or economic status does not define the person. If you are temporarily unable to work, in what ways can you be productive and contribute your current gifts at home and in the community?
   _____
   _____

*(Continued on the next page)*

INSIGHT AND EMPOWERMENT

# Major Life Activities *(continued)*

9. In your vocational life, you may be eligible for Disability Compensation. Your lawyer or advocate will focus on what you cannot do, to get the best possible benefits. Beware: although you are indeed deserving of financial remuneration for loss and suffering, afterward focus on what you *can* do. When the condition is stable and benefits are maximized, what do you want to do for the rest of your life? What talents and interests will you pursue?

   _____

10. For your life in general, you need structure and a schedule. THINGS TO DO lists and calendars keep you on track. Plan to promote physical, emotional, intellectual, social, spiritual and vocational well-being.

| Time | Sunday | Monday | Tuesday | Wednesday | Thursday | Friday | Saturday |
|---|---|---|---|---|---|---|---|
| Morning | | | | | | | |
| Afternoon | | | | | | | |
| Evening | | | | | | | |

11. ***Disability is a matter of perception. If you can do one thing well, you're needed by someone.***
    ~ Martina Navratilova.
    What can or will you learn to do well and who will need you?

    _____
    _____

12. ***No one can make you feel inferior without your consent.*** ~ Eleanor Roosevelt.
    How will you stop consenting to negativity from others or from your self-talk?

    _____
    _____

13. ***He is able who thinks he is able.*** ~ Buddha.
    What are you able to do and be?

    _____
    _____

14. ***Once I knew only darkness and stillness…My life was without past or future…But, a little word from the fingers of another fell into my hand that clutched at emptiness and my heart leaped to the rapture of living.*** ~ Helen Keller
    You may not be blind, deaf and unable to speak, but you can receive a word from another person, source, or from yourself that leads you to leap into living. What does Keller's message say to you, and how are you going to live?

    _____
    _____

# Vocational Rehabilitation Facilitator's Guide

## Measurable Behavioral Objectives

**Veterans will …**
- Identify resources for education, employment, training and other services for veterans with and without disabling conditions.
- If applicable, apply for Veteran's Rehabilitation and Employment services.
- Perform checklist ratings regarding readiness factors.
- Determine reasons to work.
- Identify loved activities and link them to occupations.
- Identify labor market information and career resources.
- Rate a prospective career regarding their needs and opportunities.
- Apply a quotation about the value of work to their lives and vocations.

## Introduction

1. Before the session begins, read this guide and the reproducible pages.
2. Decide on one of the interactive variations or the traditional approach (below).
3. Photocopy the reproducible pages but retain them until after the introduction.
4. Put the question *Why Work?* on the board and encourage participants to brainstorm.
5. A volunteer lists ideas on the board. Elicit needs in addition to financial such as belonging to a work group of people with similar interests, self esteem when mastering tasks, etc.
6. Explain there are many resources for employment and training for veterans with or without disabling conditions.

## Activity

1. Distribute the reproducible pages.
2. Take turns reading the Education and Assessment portion aloud.
3. Allow time to complete the written Insight and Empowerment questions.
4. Encourage participants to share their responses through number 5.

## Conclusion

- Encourage participants to share their responses to the quotation (number 6).

## Interactive Variations

- Ask participants to take turns reading the Insight and Empowerment questions aloud and answering orally.
- Ask participants to pair up with peers, read the questions to each other, record their partner's responses, and share with the group if they wish.

EDUCATION AND ASSESSMENT & INSIGHT AND EMPOWERMENT

# Vocational Rehabilitation

## Education and Assessment

Finances are first on the minds of many veterans. Some veterans are fortunate and can return to their prior civilian jobs. Most do not have employment waiting for them.

- If you enlisted, young, and with little job experience, your military training may relate to occupations stateside. If not, you might explore the GI Bill for education.
- The US Department of Labor's Veterans Employment and Training Services VETS Programs have Hiring Heroes and other services.
- Additionally, help with finances is available to veterans.

### If you have a disability

You may have returned a different person, with an emotional or physical impairment that affects your ability to work. You may contact the Department of Veterans Affairs regarding a service connected disability, be evaluated and given a percentage of disability rating, and apply for disability compensation. This helps your financial needs but eventually you will probably need more money and other benefits of work.

When you are stable enough emotionally and physically, explore the governmental and military information.

Check items related to your needs:
- ❏ Prepare a resume and cover letter.
- ❏ Evaluate my interests, aptitudes and abilities.
- ❏ Determine transferrable skills and experience related to the current labor market.
- ❏ Seek referrals to employers who have incentives to hire veterans.
- ❏ Accept assistance with adaptations and accommodations.
- ❏ Use entitlements to education at colleges, vocational, technical or business school.
- ❏ Match my abilities with the physical and mental demands of prospective careers.

## Insight and Empowerment

### Know Yourself.

With agencies, there will be waiting phases and delays. You can do much to prepare for your appointments and for your future. Knowing what you want is essential.

1. First, find out if you have a disability and be in the best emotional and physical shape possible.
   Check the items that you have completed:
   - ❏ A medical and psychiatric exam to determine if a disability is present
   - ❏ An idea of what you cannot do (heavy lifting? undergoing stress from the public? sensitivity to loud noises?)
   - ❏ An idea of what you can do (wheel chair administrative work? help others?)

*(Continued on the next page)*

## INSIGHT AND EMPOWERMENT

# Vocational Rehabilitation *(Continued)*

2. Work fulfills many needs. Financially it helps with food, clothing, shelter, health insurance; socially, it provides a sense of belonging to a group of people with similar interests; emotionally it helps self esteem with skills and advancement; at its highest level, values are fulfilled through creativity and helping people. You may have different motivations for working.

   a. _____
   b. _____
   c. _____
   d. _____
   e. _____

3. According to Confucius: ***Find a job you love and you'll never work a day in your life.***
   What top five things, not necessarily work related, do you love to do?

   a. _____
   b. _____
   c. _____
   d. _____
   e. _____

4. How could each become an occupation with further training or help in setting up your own business? (Remember Mrs. Fields who turned cookie baking into a business?)

   _____
   _____
   _____
   _____
   _____

## Know the Labor Market

5. Gather research for at least one occupation you like. Use the free online U.S. Department of Labor's Occupational Outlook Handbook and Career Guide to Industries, your local Employment Development Department, classified ads, and other resources. Answer the following:

   a. The pay range _____
   b. Entry level education _____
   c. Physical and emotional demands _____
   d. Future need or growth rate _____
   e. Local opportunities or your relocation considerations _____

6. Consider this quotation by Martin Luther King:

   *If a man is called to be a street sweeper, he should sweep streets even as Michelangelo painted, or Beethoven composed music, or Shakespeare composed poetry. He should sweep streets so well that all the hosts of heaven and earth will pause to say, here lived a great street sweeper who did his job well.*

   Apply the above concept to your work and your life:
   _____
   _____

# Resources

*"What's right about America is that although we have a mess of problems, we have great capacity – intellect – and resources – to do something about them."*

~ Henry Ford II

Websites, books, and Internet search topics are suggested in this section. The U.S. Department of Defense and Department of Veterans Affairs, plus many excellent military resources are listed; military and non-military mental health, addiction recovery, vocational rehabilitation, family assistance and other agencies are included. Information is provided concerning suicide prevention websites and telephone crisis lines.

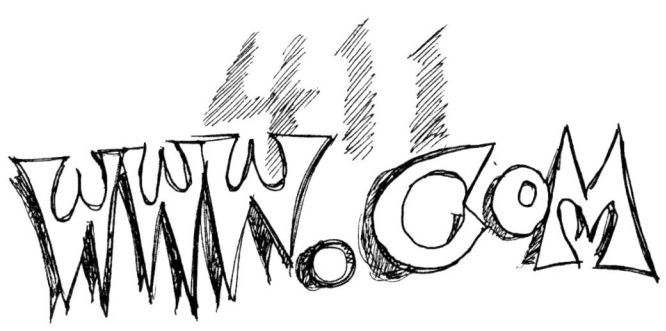

# Website Resources for Veterans

- **The American Psychiatric Association** – mental health information and advocacy.
- **The American Red Cross** – www.redcross.org comforts service members and families.
- **The American Association of Suicidology** – fact sheets and other services.
- **The American Psychological Association** – www.apa.org and other resources – types of therapy and information about finding counselors and therapists.
- **County Veteran Service Officers, Family Readiness Groups (FRG) and Family Assistance Centers (FAC)** – www.guardfamily.org – help with family issues.
- **Defense Centers of Excellence (DCoE)** – www.dcoe.health.mil – outreach; National Resource Directory searches by city, state or zip code regarding benefits, education, employment, health, housing, volunteer opportunities and other services; resources for psychological health and traumatic brain injury; Veterans Crisis Line and live chats.
- **Department of Defense** – Military Health System – (MHS) www.health.mil – finding the right mental health provider; getting the PTSD Coach mobile application; mental and physical health.
- **GI Bill** – www.gibill.gov – education and tuition assistance.
- **GI Rights Hotline** – www.girightshotline.org – non-profit, non-governmental help with complaints and rights.
- **Make the Connection** – www.maketheconnection.net – VA public awareness campaign; veterans and families find resources, health information and encouragement from veterans who have overcome obstacles.
- **Military Homefront** – www.militaryhomefront.dod.mil – help with a transition plan when leaving military service and other assistance.
- **Military One Source** – www.militaryonesource.mil – military life, family, recreation, health, relationships, financial, legal, grief and loss, crisis, disasters, domestic abuse and other issues; toll free 800 numbers for a consultant are provided.
- **National Association of County Veteran Service Officers** – www.nacvso.org claims processing and transition from military to civilian life.
- **National Institute of Mental Health** – information about PTSD and other issues.
- **National Alliance on Mental Illness (NAMI)** – www.nami.org– Veterans Resources include PTSD, depression, homelessness assistance and other information.
- **National Center for PTSD** – www.ptsd.va.gov.– booklet Understanding PTSD, available online; symptoms, how to get help, Mental Health Services Locator and a VA PTSD Program Locator. Their website provides information on managing trauma-related anger, marital and other issues.
- **National Institute on Drug Abuse** – www.drugabuse.gov – articles about veterans and families, the science of addiction and related subjects.
- **National Suicide Prevention Life-Line and the Veteran's Crisis Line** – http://www.suicidepreventionlifeline.org – 1-800-273-8255, (TALK) – crisis intervention, information, where and how to get further help.
- **Substance Abuse and Mental Health Services Administration (SAMHSA)**– www.samhsa.gov– deployment's impact on substance abuse and emotions; assessment and treatment information; invisible wounds; predicting immediate and long term consequences of mental health problems.
- **U.S. Department of Veterans Affairs** – www.va.gov – information, assistance, some applications online regarding health, prescriptions, benefits, careers, vocational rehabilitation and training; additionally the V.A. website offers links regarding home loans, adaptive sports, and help for returning service members, etc. Help with locating a chaplain is available.
- **U.S. Bureau of Labor Statistics** – www.bls.gov – The Occupational Outlook Handbook, research occupations, their expected growth, pay, level of education required, on the job training and other data; they also publish a Career Guide to Industries.
- **United Way** – www.united.org – local services for veterans and families.
- **Veterans Centers** – www.vetcenter.va.gov – geographic directory for emotional and other help.
- **Veterans Service Organizations** – www.va.gov-directory of organizations serving veterans.

# Books for Veterans and Families

- ***Welcome Them Home, Help Them Heal*** (Sippola, Blumenshine, Tubesing, Yancey) – Addresses the physical, psychological and spiritual wounds of war and sparks a spirit of willingness and hope. Post-deployment and re-deployment difficulties; healing soul wounds and violated consciences, and other problems are encompassed; circles of care are suggested; spiritual and civilian sources of help are identified.

- ***GriefWork - Healing from Loss*** (Leutenberg and Zamore) – For the facilitator. Addresses shock, disorganization, reorganization and a New Normal; deals with sorrow, expressing feelings, developing support systems.

- ***The GriefWork Companion ~ Activities for Healing*** (Leutenberg and Zamore) — For individuals. Provides self-help exercises to help survivors accept, adjust and move forward.

- ***GriefWork for Teens – Healing from Loss*** (Leutenberg and Zamore) – For facilitators of teenagers. Addresses shock, disorganization, reorganization and a New Normal; deals with sorrow, expressing feelings, developing support systems.

- ***The Complete Caregiver Support Workbook – A Reproducible Workbook for Groups and Individuals*** (Leutenberg and Morris) – Provides insight, problem solving, and ideas for starting and leading a caregiver support group as well as as a resource tool for individuals. It emphasizes self care, communication, family and close friend dynamics, advocacy, home safety and other issues.

- ***Motivation*** – Identifying strengths, interests, abilities, hopes and dreams (Leutenberg and Butler) - Provides motivation for participants to face difficulties and change, and reach their maximum potentials.

- ***Creating a Healthy Balanced Life*** (Leutenberg and Negley) – Provides reproducible activities and handouts for facilitating individual or group sessions on living a healthy, balanced life. Chapters include: The Mind, Body and Soul, Attitude, Stress-Less, Relationships and Leisure/Recreation/Play.

- ***Invisible Heroes: Survivors of Trauma and How They Heal*** (Naparstek) – This book explains why imagery is truly a key to healing. Filled with the voices of scores of actual survivors and therapists, it offers a spate of imagery know-how, a step-by-step program with more than 20 imagery scripts, tailored to the three stages of recovery, and a practical guide to the best of the new imagery-based therapies.

- ***Veterans – Surviving and Thriving after Trauma – A Reproducible Workbook Created for Facilitators to use with Returning Veterans and Their Families*** (Leutenberg and Butler) – Provides educational, assessment, insight and empowerment activities to help veterans and families face reintegration and physical, emotional, vocational and other challenges. Chapters include: Homecoming, Stress, Anger, Depression, Guilt, Grief, Substance Abuse, Coping Skills, Relationships, Rebounding and Resources.

# Additional Internet Search Topics

- **Cognitive Behavioral Therapy for Veterans** – reducing anger, stress, guilt; improving mood.
- **Disabled Veterans and Newly Disabled** – financial assistance, emotional and physical coping.
- **Guided Imagery** – Belleruth Naparstek, LISW, BCD, works with traumatized veterans.
- **Faith-Based Help for Veterans** – MyHealtheVetSpirituality Center and other resources.
- **Humana and Tricare** – military health care plans; whether or not you are covered under these plans, access information regarding emotions, children, teens, suicide myths and facts, etc.
- **Humor for Veterans** – military jokes and resources for those veterans who find humor helpful.
- **International War Veterans' Poetry Archives** – writings by war veterans and their families.
- **In-Vitro Fertilization for Veterans** – information on what is covered, recent and upcoming legislation.
- **MASH** – situation comedy, dark comedy; originally broadcast in the 1970s and early 1980s. Watching on DVD, cable TV classics, or online may help some veterans.
- **Meditation, Mindfulness, Relaxation Techniques** – self-help for stress reduction.
- **Military Portal: Find State Resources for Veterans** – educational, employment, homeless resources and information for persons in the National Guard and Reserves.
- **Military Service Dogs, Animal Assisted Therapy** – assisting veterans with obtaining pets.
- **National Military Family Association** – relationships, children, and related information.
- **Operation Homecoming** – war-related poetry and essays and other information.
- **Positive Psychology** – articles; Comprehensive Soldier Fitness: An Overview encompassing emotional, social, physical, family and spiritual aspects and other referrals.
- **Problem Solving Therapy, Reality Therapy, Solution-Focused Brief Therapy, Rational Emotive Therapy** – treatment types and related self-help concepts.
- **Reintegration after Deployment** – military articles, peer support systems, parenting, etc.
- **Stages of Grief and Loss** – articles; Managing Grief After A Disaster; PTSD, etc.
- **Stars and Stripes newspaper**; also search for publications for your branch of the military.
- **State Department of Vocational Rehabilitation** – education, training and job seeking.
- **The Wounded Warrior Project** – services promoting well-adjusted bodies and minds; economic empowerment and engagement (staying connected with other veterans and peer mentoring); Military branches also have Wounded Warrior Programs through the Department of Defense and the Department of Veterans Affairs.
- **Types of Military Veteran Organizations** – Veterans of Foreign Wars, The American Legion, AMVETS, Disabled American Veterans, Jewish War Veterans of the USA, Catholic War Veterans and American Foreign Prisoners of War and other referrals.
- **Uniformed Services Employment and Reemployment Rights Act (USERRA)** – job rights for veterans and reservists.
- **UPS Upside** – VetFranInitiative, financial incentives to encourage franchise ownership.
- **Veterans and Anger** – causes of anger and controlling aggression.
- **Veterans and Business** – FastTrac program and others; assistance in starting business ventures.
- **Veterans and Fly Fishing** – healing waters for veterans with emotional and physical issues.
- **Veterans and Guilt** – articles and referrals to veteran centers and other resources.
- **Veterans and Jobs** – Hiring Our Heroes Campaign and others; help in securing employment.
- **Veterans and Sports** – opportunities for involvement; veterans in sports history.
- **Veterans and Writing Therapy** – therapeutic writing, poetry, publication, etc.
- **Veterans and … Creative Expression, Music, Dance, Art or Drama** – how these help veterans.
- **Veterans Volunteering** – articles; TIME's Volunteer Vets: Returning Troops Still Want to Serve.
- **Wheelchair Basketball for Veterans** – opportunities to play; inspirational articles.
- **Yellow Ribbon Program** – GI Bill, education information, suicide prevention, reintegration, etc.

# Suggestions for Veterans and/or Veterans' Families at the Facilitator's Discretion

War… Movies, Television, Books, Songs, Poems - information and entertainment resources; some veterans find these helpful; others may experience unpleasant memories. Additionally, reading war poems is cathartic and writing poetry is therapeutic. Some of the poems are graphic and facilitators might wish to read them first before recommending them to veterans.

The following list of resources was prepared by Walter Skold, MLIS.

**Poetry specific to the wars in Iraq and Afghanistan include:**

a. Bill Turner's poem, "Here, Bullet," from his publisher's page; veterans may also listen to Turner reading the poem.

b. Dunya Mikhail's poems, "The War Works Hard," "Bag of Bones," and "I was in a Hurry." Dunya Mikhail is an Iraqi-American poet.

c. Ryan Alexander's poem, "The Cat".

d. "Operation Homecoming": The Writings of War; Operation Homecoming official site.

e. Listen to NPR's Morning Edition July 4, 2007 and July 6, 2007.

f. Exile's Return, the story of one of Iraq's most important poets, by Elena Lappin, in *Slate Magazine*, June 2003.

g. "From street bards to Saddam, everyone's a poet in Iraq," by Annia Ciezadlo, in *The Christian Science Monitor*, 2004.

h. International War Veterans' Poetry Archives has thousands of poems and veterans and family members are free to submit poems and essays. An example of their *Double Tap Award For War Poetry Honour Roll* is "Memorial Day Has Come and Gone."

i. Poets Against the War, started in 2003, publishes a poem of the week and organizes protest events and poetry readings.

j. Former US Poet Laureate, Robert Pinsky, penned a letter of conscience to Mrs. Bush and wrote an excellent historical article, "Poe."

### Come to the Edge

*"Come to the edge," he said.*
*They said, "We are afraid."*
*"Come to the edge," he said.*
*They came.*
*He pushed them … and they flew.*

~ Christopher Logue

Whole Person Associates is the leading publisher
of training resources for professionals who empower
people to create and maintain healthy lifestyles.
Our creative resources will help you work effectively with
your clients in the areas of stress management,
wellness promotion, mental health and life skills.

Please visit us at our web site: **www.wholeperson.com**.
You can check out our entire line of products,
place an order, request our print catalog, and
sign up for our monthly special notifications.

**Whole Person Associates**
210 W Michigan
Duluth MN 55802
800-247-6789